THE BATTLE AGAINST BACTERIA

A fresh look

THE BATTLE AGAINST BACTERIA
A fresh look

*A history of man's fight against bacterial disease
with special reference to the development
of antibacterial drugs*

PETER BALDRY

M.B., B.S., F.R.C.P.

CAMBRIDGE UNIVERSITY PRESS

CAMBRIDGE

LONDON · NEW YORK · MELBOURNE

Published by the Syndics of the Cambridge University Press
The Pitt Building, Trumpington Street, Cambridge CB2 1RP
Bentley House, 200 Euston Road, London NW1 2DB
32 East 57th Street, New York, NY 10022, USA
296 Beaconsfield Parade, Middle Park, Melbourne 3206, Australia

First published 1965
Reprinted 1967
Translated into Norwegian 1967
Translated into Japanese 1968
This edition 1976

Library of Congress Cataloguing in Publication Data
Baldry, P. E.
The battle against bacteria.
Includes index.
1. Bacteriology, Medical–History. I. Title.
QR46.B28 1976   616.01′4′09   76–639
ISBN 0 521 21268 5
(First edition   ISBN 0 521 04092 2 hard covers
ISBN 0 521 09278 7 paperback)

Printed in Great Britain
at the
University Printing House, Cambridge
(Euan Phillips, University Printer)

To
NORMAN MATHESON
F.R.C.S., F.R.A.C.S., M.R.C.P.
*without whose encouragement this book would not
have been written*

…in the field of experiment, chance favours only the prepared mind.

LOUIS PASTEUR

CONTENTS

PREFACE TO THIS EDITION

The story recounted in these pages is a continuation of the one told in my book *The Battle Against Bacteria* which, first published in 1965, traced the events in man's fight against bacterial disease up to and including the discovery of important antibacterial substances during the first fifty years of this century.

The large number of other anti-microbial agents produced in rapid succession during the past twenty-five years, with at the same time the increasing ability of bacteria to withstand attack by many of these substances, has prompted me to have a fresh look at the subject.

It will be shown that man's many successes have stemmed from initial shrewd observations followed in most cases by tedious, painstaking and often protracted work both in the laboratories of universities and of the pharmaceutical industry. The battle, however, has by no means been one-sided and the various ingenious defence measures increasingly being adopted by bacteria have led to a situation where if man is to have any chance of containing the enemy he must learn to employ the powerful weapons at his disposal in a strategic and skilful manner.

It is hoped that this book will continue to be read with interest by members of the medical and nursing professions and also by a wide section of the general public.

My sincere thanks are due to Professor E. P. Abraham, Oxford University; Dr S. R. M. Bushby, The Wellcome Research Laboratories; Dr Naomi Datta, Royal Postgraduate Medical School, London; Dr Ian Fleming, Glaxo Laboratories; and Dr G. N. Rolinson, Beecham Pharmaceuticals, for their expert guidance.

I should like to state how grateful I am to Mr S. Watkins of The Wellcome Institute for the History of Medicine for his help in selecting many of the illustrations. My thanks are also due to Miss Kathleen Young and Mrs Margaret Jackson for their invaluable help in the preparation of the manuscript. Finally, I wish to express my appreciation to the Cambridge University Press for their unfailing helpfulness during the various stages of publication.

January 1976   P. E. B.

PREFACE TO THE FIRST EDITION

Until the end of the last century there was a great risk of dying from some microbial disease before reaching the age of forty. A large number of people succumbed in infancy or childhood and others in early adult life. Now, thanks to scientific advances made in the last fifty years, death for most people in Western countries has been deferred and they have a very good chance of enjoying their full span of years. The proportion of old people in our midst today is higher than ever before and this is largely due to the recent success in the fight against microbes. As a practising physician it has been my privilege to take part in this battle and to use some of the powerful weapons at our disposal. They have brought about such a great change in the pattern of disease that I was prompted to inquire how they were discovered, and a story so dramatic and full of such interest was revealed to me, that it is the purpose of this book to share it with others.

My sincere thanks are due to Miss K. M. Young for her invaluable help in the preparation of the manuscript and to the editorial staff of the Cambridge University Press for kindly reading the text and making many helpful suggestions. I also gratefully acknowledge the advice of Dr F. N. L. Poynter, Director and formerly Chief Librarian of the Wellcome Historical Medical Library, and Mr Alistair Warren of Messrs Alex. Cowan and Sons, Ltd.

P. E. B.

ACKNOWLEDGEMENTS

We are very grateful to all copyright holders who allowed us to reproduce their illustrations here, especially the following:

Acta Medica Scandinavica   Fig. 17

Beecham Pharmaceuticals Research Division   Figs. 48, 49, 52

Edinburgh University Student Publications Board   Fig. 26

Glaxo Laboratories Ltd   Figs. 19, 51, 57(*b*)

International Review of Cytology (Academic Press Inc.)   Fig. 23

Johns Hopkins University Press   Fig. 61

Journal of Infectious Diseases (University of Chicago Press)   Figs. 20, 58

Journal of Molecular Biology (Academic Press Inc.)   Fig. 24

A. M. Lawn, Houghton Poultry Research Station, Huntingdon   Fig. 60

Professor L. J. Ludovici   Fig. 42

Medical Microbiology (Churchill Livingstone)   Fig. 25

Professor F. O'Grady   Figs. 18, 19, 20, 50, 51, 57(*a*), 57(*b*)

Pepys Library, Magdalene College, Cambridge   Fig. 3

The Royal Society of Medicine   Fig. 6

Science (© 1969 American Association for the Advancement of Science)   Fig. 50

Simon & Schuster Inc.   Fig. 53

Society for General Microbiology Ltd   Figs. 18, 21, 22, 57(*a*)

Verlagsgessellschaft Otto Spatz   Fig. 41

The Wellcome Trustees   Figs. 1, 2, 4, 5, 7, 8, 9, 10, 11, 12, 13, 14, 15, 16, 28, 29, 30, 31, 32, 34, 35, 37, 38, 39, 40

1

THE UNKNOWN ENEMY

Mankind has always been affected by disease which at times, in the form of pestilence or plague, has spread throughout entire communities. These epidemics were originally believed to be visitations by the gods intended to punish evil doers, although the mechanism by which the wrath of the gods produced this terrible effect remained unexplained. Hippocrates, the famous Greek physician, born in 460 B.C., firmly rejected this notion. A very observant man with a clear logical mind who, during the course of a long distinguished career, formulated precepts, aphorisms and laws which have had an important influence on medical thought ever since, he believed that ill health arose from external earthly causes such as cold, sun or changing winds. He noted the effect of food, occupation and climate on the causation of disease, and one of his best known books, *Airs, Waters and Places*, deals with the influence of climate, prevailing winds, water supplies, the nature of the soil and the habits of the people, on the illnesses from which they suffered. Although time has shown that these factors are of undoubted importance, it was soon obvious that they did not afford a complete explanation of the origin and spread of disease. It had long been observed that disease could be transmitted from one person to another when in close proximity and could also be spread by clothing or objects in common use. This led physicians to postulate that disease was caused by animated particles invisible to the naked eye. This theory was clearly expressed by Varro (117–26 B.C.) when he stated that disease was caused by tiny animals which could not be seen by the naked eye but which were carried with the air through the mouth and nose into the body. Similarly the early Teutons are said to have pictured minute worm-like creatures coming out of the nostrils, eyes and ears of sick individuals and passing into the bodies of others. Thus at a very early stage man developed a concept that contagious disease was caused by invisible living things, but it was not until the invention of the microscope that the idea

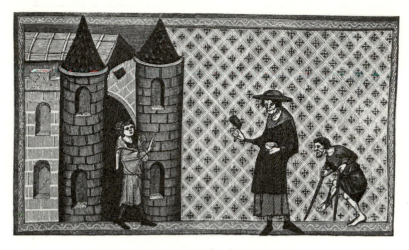

Fig. 1. Leprosarium in the thirteenth century.

could be shown to be a reality. In the meantime, however, general measures were taken to prevent the spread of contagious disease.

The ancient Hebrews recognized that leprosy was readily transmitted from one person to another and devised regulations to prevent its spread, which may be found in the thirteenth and fourteenth chapters of the book of Leviticus. Explicit instructions to be observed by the priest included the isolation of the patient, the washing and burning of infected clothing, and the disinfection of houses—if necessary their complete destruction. Strict enforcement of similar rules continued throughout many parts of the world up to the Middle Ages, so that lepers were driven out of the community away from families and friends, and forced to live in abandoned places and to subsist largely on charity. The unfortunate sufferer was made to announce his approach by shaking a bell or rattle or by blowing a horn and crying 'Unclean'. Governments also instituted compulsory medical inspection of the population and anyone deemed to be suffering from the disease was deprived of his property and pronounced legally dead. As we look back upon these practices today they appear to be

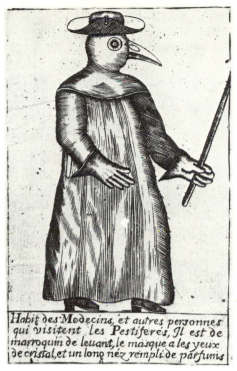

Habit des Medecins, et autres personnes qui visitent les Pestiferes, Il est de marroquin de leuant, le masque a les yeux de cristal, et un long nez rempli de parfums

Fig. 2. *Protective clothing of the kind worn by plague doctors during the seventeenth century.*

unnecessarily harsh and cruel; nevertheless, they were the first steps in public health control and did demonstrate that, in order to prevent the spread of disease in a community, it is necessary for its members to conform to certain regulations.

Plague was another disease for which rules were made to prevent its spread, long before the causative organism was recognized. It is a horrible condition which may cause large swellings in the groin and armpits, or seriously affect the lungs. The disease spread from the East and from A.D. 900 to 1500 it attacked Europe sixty-five times. The serious epidemic in the fourteenth century known as the Black Death began as usual in the Far East, where millions died in India and China, and spread to Europe in 1347, first to Italy, then to France and finally to England. In an attempt to check it in Venice

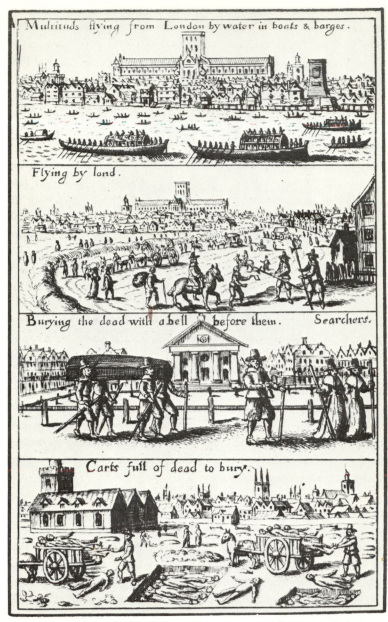

Fig. 3. Plague in the seventeenth century: scenes in London from a contemporary print in the Pepys Collection, Magdalene College, Cambridge.

a detention hospital was opened in 1403 on an island adjoining the city, for the isolation of all travellers from the Levant for a period of 30 to 40 days. The period of 40 days was apparently chosen because at that stage of world history religious ideas were dominant and that particular length of time had great biblical significance. It was from this regulation that our term 'quarantine' arose.

In 1467 a similar hospital was opened in Genoa, and in 1476 the authorities in Marseilles converted their old leper hospital into a plague hospital. By this time leprosy was so well under control that hospitals set aside for its management could be converted for use against this further health hazard. This practice of isolation and detention of travellers in order to see whether or not they were incubating the plague soon became world wide and helped to establish the general principle that transmittable diseases may be controlled by removing the sufferer from the community.

Syphilis is a further example of a disease which was known to be contagious long before the causative organism was identified. At the beginning of the sixteenth century sufficient was known about it to make diagnosis easy and, since it was realized that it was transmitted by sexual intercourse, various preventive measures could be taken to stop its spread. The disease first hit Europe with a forceful and devastating impact towards the end of the fifteenth century, when it was far more acute than at the present time. It was characterized by widespread skin eruptions and ulcers, with much destruction of tissue, which often led to death. The speed with which it reached epidemic proportions soon attracted the attention of physicians and led them to make it the subject of special study. There has been much controversy regarding the part of the world in which syphilis originated, one theory being that the sailors of Columbus, having been infected by the natives in Haiti, brought it back to the Spanish occupants of Naples. There is evidence however to show that it was in Europe before the discovery of America. A further theory is that it was brought to Europe by sailors landing on the south coast of Spain after returning from voyages to West Africa; the exact truth will probably never be known. There seems little doubt that the disease ravaged the army of Charles VIII of France during the siege of Naples in 1495 and was disseminated widely by his band of mer-

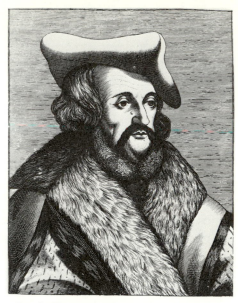

Fig. 4. Hieronymus Fracastorius (1483–1553).

cenaries on their return to France, so the French called it the
Neapolitan disease while the Spaniards always referred to it as the
French disease. It was the Italian physician Fracastorius (1483–
1553) who put an end to the argument by giving it the name of
syphilis. He was especially interested in diseases which spread from
one person to another and had made a study of leprosy and plague,
both of which by his time, as has been shown, were controlled by
isolation of the victim and destruction of contaminated objects.
When a new type of disease which seemed to be passed from one
person to another during sexual intercourse appeared in the neighbourhood, he quickly became interested. After a period of study he
became inspired to write a poem about it in Latin hexameter! Turning to Ovid to find a name for a central character his choice fell upon
Syphilus, the second son of Niobe. In his poem, Syphilus, a shepherd
boy, because of an act of impiety, brought down upon him the anger
of the sun god and was given as a punishment a loathsome and contagious disease. The poem became famous and it was from the name
of this mythical character that the disease received its title. He pub-

lished the results of his studies on these three contagious diseases, leprosy, plague and syphilis, in a famous book *De Contagione*, in 1546. He postulated that certain diseases were transmitted by imperceptible particles which he called *seminaria contagionum* or the 'seeds of disease', and considered that this could happen either by direct contact with the sick person, or by contact with his clothing or utensils, or in some cases by the 'seeds' being carried through the air. His concept was extraordinarily clear, although formulated centuries before it could be proved that certain diseases are spread by bacteria. His book was a most valuable contribution to knowledge about the control of infectious diseases and, because of it, he has the right to be regarded as the father of modern epidemiology.

In addition to passing laws about individual diseases, the human race was quick to appreciate the value of general rules of hygiene, as is again shown in the Old Testament. A good example appears in Deuteronomy, chapter xxiii, verse 13, where Moses gives instructions that every soldier shall carry a spade in order to bury his excreta so as not to defile the camp—'and thou shalt have a paddle upon thy weapon; and it shall be, when thou wilt ease thyself abroad, thou shalt dig therewith, and shalt turn back and cover that which cometh from thee'. The disposal of sewage in big towns is obviously a far more difficult problem, but unfortunately those in authority have not always been sufficiently strict in the matter. This applied in Great Britain up to the nineteenth century and is still true in certain parts of the world. Because of this lack of insistence on proper sanitation, there were serious widespread epidemics of cholera, typhoid and dysentery in Europe up to the middle of the last century. The description of conditions in big cities at that time showed that the filth was appalling. In the tenements of Glasgow dung was left lying in the courtyards adjacent to the houses as there were no drains or privies; in another Scottish town it was reported that there were no lavatories in houses and only two or three public privies, situated in the better parts of the town. These two examples were typical of the situation in all big cities. This lack of lavatories either public or private led to the habit of house dwellers filling chamber pots with excreta and after some days, when completely full, and with a shout of 'Gardez l'eau', emptying the contents out of the window into the

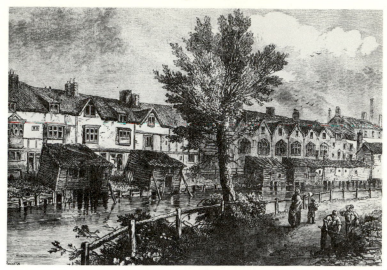

*Fig. 5. Old houses in London's Dockland around 1810. The stream was the
sole water supply and means of sewage disposal.*

street below; a habit not without risk to passers by, and of course a
practice which led to persistent pollution and stench in all the streets.
The lawyer Edwin Chadwick (1800–90) attempted to reform these
conditions, producing in 1842 the well known report on the sanitary
conditions of the labouring population in Great Britain in which he
pointed out that much disease could be prevented by proper drainage,
the removal of refuse from houses and streets, and the improvement
of water supplies.

Doubt as to whether excreta alone could cause disease however
was already present in the minds of thinking people before germs were
identified under the microscope. William Budd, the great epidemio-
logist of the nineteenth century, took the opportunity of the famous
Great Stench of London, which occurred during the summer months
of 1858, to point out that organic putrefaction by itself was not
enough to cause disease. At that time, the sewage of nearly three
million people was allowed to collect in one vast cess-pit in the middle
of the city, and during the summer the hot sun shining on this quag-
mire produced a stench so foul as had never been experienced before.
The work of Parliament was almost brought to a standstill because

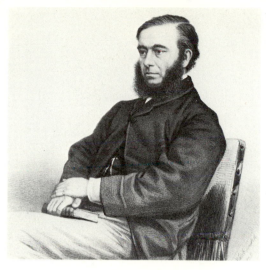

Fig. 6. William Budd (1811–80).

of the noxious air which penetrated the building, and steps were taken to overcome this by the suspension before every window of blankets saturated in chloride of lime, and by the lavish use of this and other disinfectants in every room. The Law Courts had to close down and travellers who could do so avoided London by making a wide detour of the city. The newspapers were full of letters from anxious members of the public about the stench, some prophesying calamity, others suggesting remedies; it became the most frequent topic of conversation, everyone convinced that it would be followed by a widespread and devastating epidemic of disease. People were amazed to find that as the season passed there was in fact a remarkable diminution in the proportion of fevers, diarrhoea and other forms of disease which had commonly been attributed to decaying dung. It was obvious therefore that this had to contain some additional poison to make it harmful, a fact which had already been shown to be true by some observations made by John Snow in 1854, during the last great cholera epidemic in Great Britain. He considered that cholera, a disease in which there is profuse and watery diarrhoea, was due to a poison taken into the mouth with excreta from some other sufferer. He believed that this could happen if con-

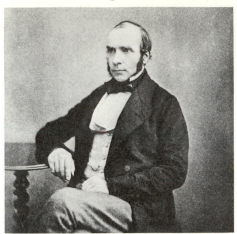

Fig. 7. John Snow (1813–58).

taminated water was used for drinking, and proved this theory by studying a large number of outbreaks and by paying special attention in every instance to the water supply. At first his teaching was ignored, until he was able to present striking supporting evidence at the time of a dramatic outbreak of the disease in Broad Street, London. In this epidemic 500 people living within two hundred yards of where the first case was diagnosed, died of the disease within the incredibly short period of ten days. The rest of the inhabitants of the street not unnaturally took fright and hurriedly left. Snow was able to show that all the victims used a pump connected to one particular well and that a person suffering from cholera had been in the habit of using a certain cesspool which he found drained into this well. As soon as he put the pump out of action by removing the handle no further case occurred. Although he was not able to demonstrate the micro-organism responsible for cholera, he established by inference that the disease is spread by water which has been contaminated by excreta containing some noxious agent.

There was therefore good evidence by the middle of the last century that some diseases are spread by air and some by water, while others like syphilis and leprosy are spread by the direct contact of one person with another. In addition it was becoming recognized that it was possible for a healthy person to be the carrier of germs and to

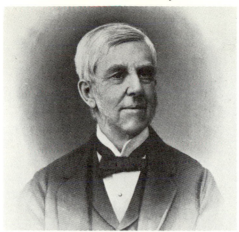

Fig. 8. Oliver Wendell Holmes (1809-94).

spread them to other people causing them to become ill. This was perhaps best demonstrated in the maternity hospitals where it was found that a very high percentage of women admitted to hospital for the birth of their babies developed an overwhelming and usually fatal form of blood poisoning some days afterwards. This feverish illness, because it occurred in the puerperium, was called puerperal fever and it is reported that out of 9886 pregnant women who were confined in the maternity hospital in Paris between 1861 and 1864, 1226 died of this disease. The situation was similarly bad in all the lying-in hospitals in Europe and other parts of the world. Oliver Wendell Holmes of Boston taught, in 1843, that puerperal fever was caused by germs on the hands of physicians and midwives carried into the bodies of these unfortunate women during internal examinations. There was much opposition to this theory, for the medical profession resented the implication that physicians were not clean, and his warning was not heeded in America for a long time. Semmelweiss taught the same principle in the maternity hospital in Vienna, but was similarly ignored. He realized that the medical students often came straight to the maternity wards after dealing with highly infectious patients in other wards, as well as after dissecting dead bodies in the post-mortem room. He therefore made it a strict rule that all students should wash their hands in a solution of chloride of lime

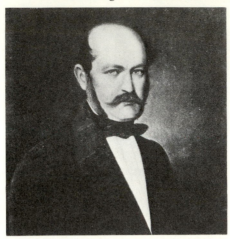

Fig. 9. Ignaz Phillipp Semmelweiss (1818–65).

before carrying out internal examinations on women, and by this means the mortality rate on his wards fell from 18 per cent to only 1 per cent. In spite of this remarkable success he was scorned, persecuted and forced to resign his position as professor, and moved to Budapest where in 1861 he published his book *The Cause and Prevention of Puerperal Fever*, but he never convinced his critics. He became insane and died from a septic wound of the hand, a tragic ending for a man whose teaching has since been proved correct.

It may be seen therefore that observant men were able to gain much knowledge about the spread and control of certain diseases long before the causative germs were identified under the microscope.

2

THE ENEMY IDENTIFIED

It is thought that a knowledge of lenses developed about the time of Euclid in the third century B.C. and that Ptolemy of Alexandria (about A.D. 150) was probably the first to study the laws of refraction of light. In England, the Franciscan friar Roger Bacon (1214–94) did much work with lenses and clearly set out the laws of refraction and reflection; he also suggested the use of lenses to improve vision. Leonardo da Vinci, in the fifteenth century, was well acquainted with the use of lenses, and Zacharias Jansen, a Dutch spectacle maker, about 1609, accidentally discovered the principle of the telescope and microscope by placing two lenses together in a tube.

The first to apply this invention to medicine was Professor Kircher (1602–80), a Jesuit priest and doctor of Würzburg. He examined the blood of patients suffering from plague, and reported that through the microscope he saw countless masses of small worms invisible to the naked eye. It has since been generally agreed that he was really only looking at red blood cells as the magnification available in his day would not have been sufficient to show the tiny germs which cause plague. Nevertheless he must be given credit for having made the correct deduction that a contagious disease was caused by microscopic organisms.

The greatest of all early microscopists was Antony Van Leeuwenhoek (1632–1723), a Dutch draper, whose interest in microscopes started as a hobby early in his life. He made a large number of them and at his death bequeathed twenty-six lenses set in silver to the Royal Society of London. He made several observations by looking down the microscope and was the first to show that the red cells in the blood of men are round, whereas in fish and amphibians they are oval. He also described many of the microscopic organisms seen in stagnant pond life but his most important achievement, from the medical point of view, was that he was the first to see the little animalcules, as he called them, which cause disease. His demonstrations

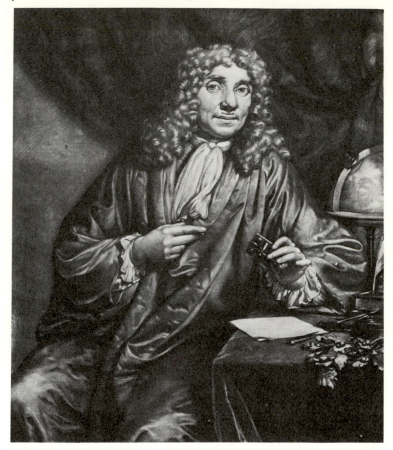

Fig. 10. Antony Van Leeuwenhoek (1632–1723).

of bacteria were made public by letters to the Royal Society between 1675 and 1685. He made detailed observations of the bacteria to be found in the mouth by examining the deposit which collected round his teeth and he said that he saw 'little animals more numerous than all the people in the Netherlands and moving about in the most delightful manner'. Although many people at that time considered that animalcules such as Leeuwenhoek described might well be the cause of contagious disease, it was not for another two hundred years that this idea was finally accepted and firmly established as a scientific fact.

Marcus Plenciz, a Viennese physician, in his *Opera Medico-*

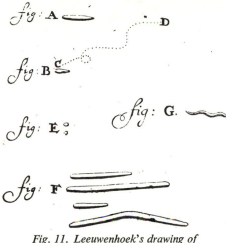

Fig. 11. *Leeuwenhoek's drawing of bacteria as seen by him.*

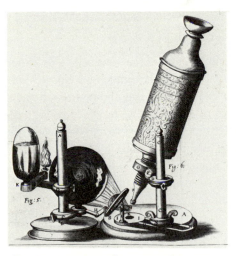

Fig. 12. *A seventeenth-century microscope.*

Physica published in 1762, clearly expressed the opinion that infectious diseases were spread through the air by contagious animalcules, though he was unable to put forward any proof of this. Probably the first man to present real evidence that living organisms were the cause of disease was Bassi, who in 1836, after working for years on a

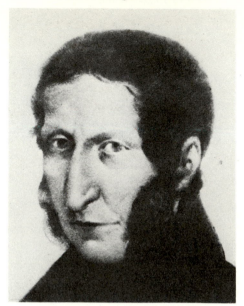

Fig. 13. Agostino Bassi (1773–1856).

certain disease which affects silkworms, was able to demonstrate that it was caused by a fungus which could be transmitted from one worm to another. No definite evidence about the part played by bacteria in the production of disease could however be obtained until a large number of different micro-organisms had been identified. An important contribution to this was made by Ehrenberg (1795–1876), who was able to distinguish between various types of micro-organisms and to place them in a simple classification. His task was made easier by using a technique, introduced by Wilhelm von Gleichen, of staining the organisms with powdered carmine or indigo. Scientists sought hard to find microbes in diseased tissue in order to be able to prove the microbial cause of infective disease, but many were carried away by their enthusiasm and made rash statements based on slipshod and uncritical work. This led the anatomist Jacob Henle to write an essay in 1840 in which he protested vigorously against certain ill-founded conclusions. He stated that before any microscopic organism could be regarded as a cause of disease in man, it must be found constantly in the diseased tissue, it must be isolated from it, and it must be possible to reproduce the disease with it. These clear principles were to influence greatly two men, Louis Pasteur and Robert Koch, who twenty years later were able to place the germ theory of disease on a sound scientific basis.

Louis Pasteur came from a humble home. His father, who had been a sergeant in Napoleon's army, was working as a tanner in the little town of Dole in Southern France when Louis was born in 1822. He was a conscientious lad, but there was nothing to make him stand out from others except, in his teens, a proficiency in portrait painting and, as a student, a determination that one day he would become a professor himself. After he qualified he asked the famous chemist Jean Dumas to employ him as a teaching assistant because, as he said, he had the ambition to become a distinguished professor; to a friend he wrote 'those of us who are to become professors must make the art of teaching our chief concern'—an extremely praiseworthy attitude, all too often lacking in men of great academic attainment. He proved himself to be an excellent teacher, but was not content merely to pass on knowledge obtained by others; he also had an innate drive to make original discoveries.

He was fortunate as a student in having the stimulating influence of two great chemists, Dumas and Antoine Balard. Dumas, a dynamic teacher, was to remain an inspiration to Pasteur all his life. Balard was a colourful, if somewhat eccentric, chemist who, even after he achieved success, lived in a shabby room furnished with two shaky armchairs which he painted a peculiar red colour under the illusion that it made them look as if they were made of mahogany! He was nevertheless a man of great ability, who took a deep personal interest in his student, and encouraged him to spend his spare time doing chemical experiments in his laboratory. Pasteur took good advantage of this and it was there that before long he made important fundamental contributions to the science of crystallography.

After Pasteur passed his examinations his tutors were very anxious for him to stay in Paris, but a decision was made by the Minister of Education to send him elsewhere to take up a teaching post. First, he was given a junior post at Dijon in 1847, but after a few months he was sent as acting professor of chemistry at the University of Strasbourg. This was a happy choice because it brought him into contact with Pierre Bertin-Mourot, professor of physics at the University in whose house he stayed. This physicist was not only an able scientist and teacher, but also had a great capacity to enjoy life, and introduced the serious-minded, intense, humourless young scholar to some of the simple pleasures of living, inculcating in him an appreciation of good wine and beer, which surprisingly enough, as will be seen, was to be a great asset to him before long in his professional life. It was also at Strasbourg that he met Marie Laurent, the daughter of the university rector, who was to share a long and happy life with him after their marriage in 1849. Pasteur's approach to the gentleman whose daughter he wished to marry was simple and direct; he wrote to him explaining that he had no money, but was imbued with good health, courage and a position in the university. He added that he had held a doctor's degree for eighteen months and had presented a few pieces of original work to the Academy of Science which had been well received. He then took the somewhat unusual step, for a suitor seeking to commend himself to a prospective father-in-law, of enclosing a report of an investigation which he had recently presented to a learned society!

The course of his life was again changed by a decree of the Minister of Education, when in 1854 he was appointed professor of chemistry at Lille, with the recommendation that he centred his teaching and research round the problems of the local industries. One of the main industries in this city was the fermentation of beet sugar to produce alcohol, and surprisingly, it was a study of this that led Pasteur to an understanding of the part played by microbes in the production of disease. Shortly after arriving at Lille he was asked to investigate certain difficulties experienced in this particular industry which led Marie Pasteur to complain, in a letter to her father, that 'Louis spends all his days in the distillery and is up to his neck in beet juice!'

The term fermentation was used in those days to describe the process by which spiritous or acid substances were obtained from organic liquids, but it was not known how this took place. Thus the production of alcohol from beet juice was called alcoholic fermentation; the conversion of wine into vinegar was called acetic acid fermentation; and the souring of milk, during which lactic acid is produced, was called lactic acid fermentation. It was thought that the fermentation of liquids was possibly brought about by changes similar to those which occurred in meat or eggs during decomposition and putrefaction. The great chemists of that time, such as Lavoisier, Gay-Lussac, Thénard and Dumas, taught that all changes in organic substances could be readily explained in terms of chemical reactions and expressed by means of chemical formulae. Lavoisier was therefore content to explain the production of alcohol from carbohydrate by stating that the latter split into two parts and that, by transfer of oxygen from one part to another, alcohol was formed. This failed to explain what made the carbohydrate undergo this change, and also ignored the fact that yeast always had to be present for it to take place. This substance had been known since primitive man used it not only to change starch into bread, but also to produce alcoholic liquids from sugar solutions.

In the 1830's it was shown that yeast was not simply an organic substance, but was made up of living cells which, under the microscope, could be observed to multiply by budding. Many people considered that alcoholic fermentation must depend on the presence and action of these living cells, but the leading chemists, including Liebig, did everything possible to discredit this theory. Liebig was willing to concede that yeast may be a small plant, but considered that, if it made any contribution to alcoholic fermentation, it was not during life, but only after death, when its protein imparted a vibration to the sugar molecule causing it to break down, with the production of alcohol. As Pasteur had been trained as a chemist it would have been easy for him to conform to these current orthodox opinions, but to his eternal credit he would not be dominated by his teachers and, seeing the weakness in their theories, was determined to discover the truth. He confirmed, by well designed experiments, that the production of alcohol from sugar was brought about by the action of yeast cells and that the amount of alcohol produced was directly proportional to the number of cells present. He had previously shown that a grey material, made out of living cells which were smaller but otherwise similar to yeast cells, was sometimes found in milk, and that this material acted as a ferment turning the milk sour with the production of lactic acid.

He next studied the manufacture of vinegar. It was well known that vinegar was produced by the oxidation of alcohol, a process which at that time was considered to be purely chemical. In France, alcohol was allowed to undergo this oxidation in casks standing on end, while the German process consisted of pouring a mixture of alcohol, acetic acid and beer over a hollow column, several metres high, of loosely piled beech shavings. These two well-known processes had been devised many years previously in an empirical manner without anyone knowing why they worked, although Liebig considered he could explain the mechanism in both cases on the basis of organic chemical reactions. He ignored however the fact that the French workers in Orleans had observed that a fragile skin or pellicle always formed on the surface of the liquid in the casks, and that for the change from wine to vinegar to take place this pellicle had to remain intact. It was for this reason that the skin was known as 'the mother of vinegar'. When in 1837 Kützing demonstrated that it was made up of living cells, some people concluded that these cells must be responsible for the essential chemical change. The chemists were not willing to consider this idea, but Pasteur felt it was worth further investigation, and was able to prove in the laboratory that the microscopic cells present in the thin skin covering the wine were responsible for its conversion into vinegar. He was also able to detect a barely visible film of organisms on the surface of the wood shavings used in the German process, and showed that if these shavings were heated, the organisms were destroyed and the shavings were then useless for their purpose. He was thus able to supply a clear explanation for this well established technique and to recommend certain alterations which enabled the manufacture of vinegar to become more efficient.

Pasteur's work on the production of lactic acid, alcohol and vinegar was of great fundamental importance for, from this, scientists had to accept that changes in organic material could be brought about by microscopic organisms.

His next step was to demonstrate the adverse effect which certain microbes could have on the fermentation of wine and beer. He published his findings in a book about wine in 1866. His interest in the subject started while he was on holiday at Arbois in 1858, for it was there that he examined samples of Jura wines under the microscope and saw living cells in them similar to the lactic acid organisms he had observed in sour milk. This observation, together with his experiments in the distilleries, led him to conclude that fermentation of wine could be disturbed by other organisms competing with yeast. A friend at Arbois then asked him to examine microscopically a selection of good and sour wines and he was able to demonstrate various micro-organisms amongst the yeast cells in the spoiled wine, whereas in the good wine he found the yeast cells alone without any additional bacteria. He was thus able to demonstrate that wine will go sour if it contains organisms other than yeast.

In 1877 Pasteur published a book in which he showed that deterioration of beer also occurs if foreign bacteria are present. He described how, when he was invited to one of the large London breweries in 1871, he took his microscope with him, and in the presence of the managers, examined a sample of their yeast used to make porter. He decided that, since he saw other micro-organisms amongst the yeast cells, the porter was probably not satisfactory, and was pleased to find that the brewers did not disagree. He then studied the yeast used to make other types of beer and found them similarly contaminated. Next, he was asked to examine under the microscope one sample of beer which was cloudy and another which was clear, and quickly recognized a large number of bacteria in the cloudy sample, but also, after careful examination, found a few in the clear one. From this he concluded that both samples would rapidly spoil and were even then not at their best: to this everyone present had somewhat reluctantly to agree.

As bacteria could spoil wine and beer, it was obvious to Pasteur that it was essential to avoid introducing them during manufacture, or to kill them if already present. He realized that, even by the most careful technique of preparation, it would be impossible to avoid a few gaining entry, which would then multiply, so that the only practical method would be to kill any organisms after they had been introduced. He appreciated that this could be achieved by heat, but also knew that excessive heat would spoil the wine, so he tried the effect of adding various chemicals, but without success. He then developed a process of rapid heating to only about 55° C, out of contact with air, and found that this was sufficient to kill the bacteria, without spoiling the wine. This process soon became known throughout the world as pasteurization and has been used ever since for the preservation of wine, beer and milk.

Before the Renaissance, it was generally believed that plants and animals could, in certain circumstances, be created from any inanimate matter. This possibility is mentioned by several early writers, including Aristotle (384–322 B.C.), and as late as the sixteenth century Van Helmont (1577–1644), a celebrated chemist, reported that one could create mice at will by placing some dirty linen together with a piece of cheese in a container! In the seventeenth century it was still thought that plants and certain small creatures such as flies, ants, spiders and other insects were produced by abiogenesis. This was challenged by Francesco Redi (1626–97) who conducted experiments to show that this theory of spontaneous generation was untrue, at least for animals large enough to be seen with the naked eye. It remained however the general opinion that the living organisms of microscopic size found in large numbers in decaying organic material were produced by a chemical reaction and thus by a form of spontaneous generation. This theory was supported by the testimony of a Catholic priest, John Needham (1713–81), who stated that he had observed the spontaneous creation of living microscopic organisms, but it was refuted by the Italian anatomist, Spallanzani (1729–99) who conducted experiments to show that it was impossible.

It was well recognized that putrefaction in organic matter could be prevented by heating it to a high temperature, so that any microbes present would be killed; also that, provided it was then protected from the air, no further microbes would appear in it; but that if it was exposed to the air they would reappear. Those who believed that these microbes developed by spontaneous generation, inferred from these observations that this process would only occur in the presence of oxygen. Others realized that a more likely explanation was that the microbes were already present in the air and were deposited on the substance. This controversy raged fiercely until Louis Pasteur finally produced evidence to solve the problem. Several people tried to prove him wrong but, by his expert technique, with close attention to detail, they were eventually silenced. He not only solved this particular dispute but, in the course of his experiments, established proper methods of working with micro-organisms which had not been adopted previously.

He first demonstrated the presence of bacteria in the air by drawing air through a tube plugged by a cotton-wool filter. The dust which collected in this filter was then examined and found to contain numerous microscopic organisms. When this dust was sprinkled on to an organic substance, previously heated to kill off bacteria in it, and kept in a vacuum, there was a rapid growth of micro-organisms. There could therefore be no doubt that these micro-organisms had been present in the dust from the air, and it has since been shown that air is in fact an important carrier of bacteria harmful to man.

One of the experiments which Pasteur conducted on this subject will remain a classic for all time. He took a number of flasks filled with a liquid containing yeast and sugar, drew out the neck of each flask to a fine point by heating it in a flame, and then boiled the liquid to drive out the air and destroy anything living in it. The flasks were then sealed off completely by heating the drawn-out ends with a blowpipe. They were now free of living material and, because of this, remained sterile for as long as they were kept sealed. He placed them in widely differing types of geographical location, and then broke the neck of each with a long pair of pincers so as to allow the introduction of air. This had to be done with the utmost care and attention to detail: the neck of the flask and the pincers had first to be heated to kill all bacteria on them, and he had to be careful to break the glass with the pincers held well above his head so that the air was not contaminated with dust from his clothes. Once the neck of a flask was broken the surrounding air surged in to fill the vacuum already created, and each flask was then resealed in a flame. Some of them remained sterile while others developed a profuse growth of bacteria. He showed from these experiments that bacteria were either absent or few in number in the high mountainous districts, but plentiful in low-lying ground. At the same time he was able to produce irrefutable proof that microbes will not appear in an organic substance when it is exposed to air, unless they are already present in the air. It is important to note that Pasteur took great care to see that there was no contamination of the flasks to spoil his experiment, and that he achieved this by sterilizing the instruments and apparatus

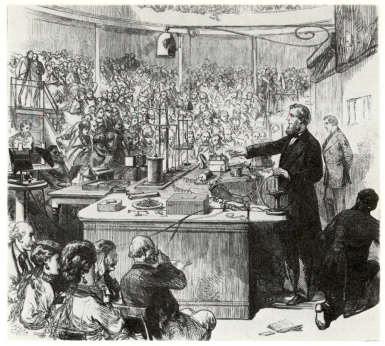

Fig. 14. John Tyndall (1820–93) lecturing at the Royal Institution.

by heat—a method which has been adopted by bacteriologists ever since. The arguments about the possibility of spontaneous generation would never have raged so fiercely or for so long, if other workers in his day had been as careful. It should be mentioned that the English physicist, John Tyndall, also deserves credit for helping to lay the ghost of spontaneous generation by his experiments, of which accounts were published in 1876 and 1877 and, together with some other lectures, in a book entitled *Essays on the floating matter of the air in relation to putrefaction and infection*, issued in 1881. These experiments confirmed Pasteur's findings in every way.

Another of Pasteur's important investigations was into diseases which affect silkworms. The knowledge gained about the behaviour of disease-producing bacteria and the control of epidemics in these insects, was to prove extremely useful to him when he later studied the part played by micro-organisms in diseases which affect man.

It may be recalled that, by a strange coincidence, it had also been work on silkworms that led the Italian, Agostino Bassi (1773–1856) to confirm for the first time that disease can be caused by living micro-organisms. Now, in the middle of the nineteenth century, just about the time of Bassi's death, silkworms were again decimated by disease to such an extent that the industry in France was on the verge of ruin, and the epidemic had spread to Italy, Spain and Austria, eventually affecting the industry in Greece, Turkey, China and Japan. Pasteur was asked by the French Minister of Agriculture to study the problem and began his investigation in 1865, knowing nothing of the habits of silkworms, and little about any micro-organisms which might infect them. He applied himself assiduously to the problem but it was five years before he reached a solution. The first two years of the study were marred by personal sorrow; in the first year his father died and this was followed later in the year by the death of his two-year-old daughter. The following year he was to suffer the loss of another daughter at the age of twelve from typhoid fever—a poignant reminder of the frequency with which parents had to face the death of children in the days before bacterial infections could be controlled.

During the course of the next three years, he was helped in the investigation by his wife and one surviving daughter, and eventually was able to show how certain diseases in silkworms could be avoided. It was time well spent because he was not only able to bring back prosperity to the industry in France but, perhaps of more importance, he acquired basic knowledge which was to prove of great value when he came to study disease in higher animals and man a few years later. He appreciated this himself, and advised those who came to help him in later years to read about his investigations into silkworms, as he believed this would give them a good introduction to this type of work.

Pasteur's work, including his studies into fermentation, his observations on the effect of micro-organisms in milk, beer and wine, and his epidemiological studies into diseases which affect silkworms, played an important part in leading doctors to consider the possibility that some diseases which affect human beings might also be brought about by microbes. This idea was not however readily accepted, as it seemed unreasonable to some people that disease in man could be brought about by minute living particles. It was accepted that microscopic organisms were found in diseased or dead tissue, but it was considered that they were more likely to be secondary invaders than the actual cause of the disease. Obermeier in 1868 reported that he had constantly found large numbers of spiral shaped organisms in blood of patients suffering from a disease called relapsing fever. It has in fact been confirmed since then that these particular microbes are the cause of this condition, but the discovery of organisms in the blood of a patient with a disease is not sufficient to prove that the disease is caused by the organisms, without further supporting evidence. Many people believed that, once the body became diseased, micro-organisms could appear in the affected tissue *de novo*, whilst others thought that tissues devitalized by disease were more prone to secondary invasion by micro-organisms entering the body from outside. It was therefore necessary, in order to prove that a disease was caused by certain specific organisms, for someone to show that, not only were they constantly present in this disease, but that they could be isolated and were then capable of reproducing the disease in another animal. The first man to supply such evidence was Robert Koch.

3

THE ENEMY NAMED

Robert Koch (1843–1910) showed an interest in science from an early age and, under the guidance of his father, became a proficient geologist, botanist and zoologist, so that gradually, during his early years, he acquired an extensive collection of minerals, plants and animals. On leaving school he entered the University of Göttingen to study medicine. He was an able student who made the most of every opportunity. At the same time he was extremely fortunate in his teachers. His professor of anatomy was Jacob Henle, the man who laid down important criteria which he insisted should be fulfilled before any specific organisms could be accepted as the cause of a given disease. He also came under the influence of the famous pathologist Krause and, as his assistant, gained useful experience, including a thorough knowledge of the technique of microscopy.

After qualification in 1866 he held junior posts in hospitals at Hanover and Hamburg and then entered general practice. His career was interrupted by the Franco-Prussian war in which he served as an army surgeon. When this was over, he found he could not settle down again to the life of a general practitioner, so studied for a higher examination in medicine, which he passed in 1872. After this he worked as a physician at Wollstein in East Prussia, where he soon built up a busy and lucrative consultant practice. He bought expensive apparatus, including a microscope and equipment to carry out photomicrography, which he installed in a laboratory next door to his consulting room. During the next four years, in addition to his clinical work, he made a special study of the disease called anthrax which was particularly prevalent amongst both animals and man in his community. Repeated examinations of the blood and tissues of affected animals showed the presence of a certain type of bacterium which he managed to isolate and study outside the body. He was then able to inject the organism into mice, guinea-pigs and rabbits, and to produce a similar disease in them. This was the first time that

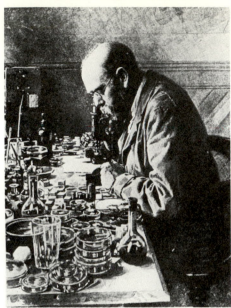

Fig. 15. Robert Koch (1843–1910).

an organism isolated from damaged tissue had been cultured in the laboratory and then used to infect another animal. It was an important landmark in the history of bacteriology, and the work was accepted by everybody, except a Frenchman called Paul Bert (1833–86) who conducted experiments designed to show that Koch's conclusions were wrong. The challenge was taken up by Louis Pasteur who hastened to the assistance of Koch, and who, by well designed and meticulously executed experiments, was able to support him in his views. It was from the evidence thus produced by Koch and Pasteur that the germ theory of disease became universally accepted.

It was now essential to study the characteristics of the various types of micro-organisms so that they could be separately named and divided into groups. German bacteriologists had made many limited attempts to do this but the first reasonably accurate and worthwhile classification was made by Ferdinand Cohn in 1872. He was handicapped however by a lack of knowledge of techniques for staining bacteria; these were later developed by Robert Koch and enabled

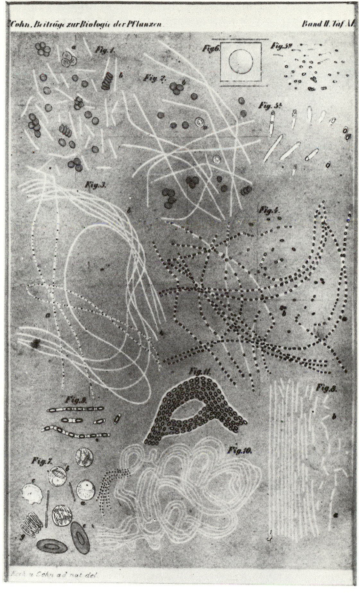

Fig. 16. The anthrax bacillus. The illustration is taken from
a paper by Robert Koch published in 1876.

him to make some of the most important contributions to this subject. Simple dyes had been used to stain bacteria for some time, but Koch was the first man to use the newly discovered aniline dyes for this purpose. These are very powerful and he found they readily adhered to bacteria, making them stand out prominently under the microscope. He also developed a method of photomicrography which helped him considerably in this work.

In 1880 Koch was appointed to work in the laboratories at Bonn University where, with the help of enthusiastic assistants, he soon published important advances in bacteriological technique. In order to study bacteria in the laboratory they must be cultured on special nutrient substances. Up to that time fluids such as broth or blood serum had been commonly used, but Koch found it was possible—and advantageous—to use solid media which included agar, a substance derived from the stems of various seaweeds found in Japan; he also used agar enriched with blood, gelatine and solidified blood serum. These substances remain in common use today together with others introduced since that time. It was by the use of such solid culture media that he was able to establish a very important method of separating bacteria so that a pure growth of each type could be obtained. As this method is still employed in routine laboratory work it will be described in detail.

A piece of wire bent to form a loop at one end is first heated to kill any bacteria adherent to it and a loop full of the specimen under examination is smeared over the surface of the culture medium which is then placed in an incubator to be kept warm at body temperature, 37 °C, for about two days. At the end of this time it is found that different types of bacteria will have grown in individual clumps or colonies. A colony of each particular type has its own characteristic appearance so that a loop full of any one can then be transferred to a separate culture plate, and in this way a pure growth of each variety of bacteria present may be obtained. This simple and effective technique was a great advance, because up to that time accurate classification, with identification and naming of the particular organisms which cause different types of disease, had been seriously handicapped by inability to separate them. After this, progress was rapid and, by about the beginning of this century, scientists had identified and named most of the bacteria harmful to man.

Koch and his pupils were responsible for much of this work and he himself acquired much fame in 1882 by his discovery of the tubercle bacillus, the germ which causes tuberculosis. Most organisms grown on a culture medium produce visible colonies after incubation for about 48 hours but tubercle bacilli divide much more slowly and it is to Koch's credit that, instead of discarding his culture plates after a few days, he persevered and showed that visible colonies of these organisms could be produced after several weeks' incubation. It was from such a culture that he was able to produce tuberculosis in a number of susceptible animals.

His anatomy teacher Henle had stated in 1840 that 'before microscopic forms can be regarded as the cause of contagion in man they must be found constantly in the contagious material, they must be isolated from it and their strength tested'. Koch was able to fulfil all these criteria with the tubercle bacillus, and in an address before the International Medical Congress in Berlin in 1890 laid down even more exacting principles, now known as 'Koch's postulates', to which each different type of organism must conform before it may be regarded as the cause of a disease. First, the organism must be found in every case of the disease and under conditions which explain the pathological changes and clinical symptoms; secondly, it must not be found as an accidental organism in other diseases; thirdly, after it has been isolated from the body and cultivated in pure culture, it must have the ability to produce the disease in animals. These basic rules are given in detail to show the remarkable clarity of his approach to this subject. By his insistence on such strict criteria he dissuaded bacteriologists from too readily drawing unwarranted conclusions from their observations, but at the same time, by removing confusion, it led them to make rapid progress in the accurate identification of disease-producing organisms. It has not always proved possible to fulfil every one of Koch's postulates, but, by adhering to them as closely as possible, serious errors have been prevented. As he himself said 'as soon as the right method is found discoveries come as easily as ripe apples fall from the tree'.

After five years in Bonn he became professor of hygiene in the University of Berlin where he organized the first systematic student course in bacteriology ever to be given. A few years later, in 1891, he became Director of the Institute of Infectious Diseases in Berlin, an establishment which was built specially for him, under his direction.

In 1890 Koch reported the preparation of tuberculin which is a protein derivative of the tubercle bacillus. There is little doubt that, from the results he obtained with experiments on guinea-pigs, he thought it was possible to treat tuberculosis with this substance. Soon the news spread, by means of the public press, that Koch had found an effective treatment for this disease, and his laboratory in Berlin was immediately besieged by physicians and their patients. Tragedy and disillusionment were to follow, as none of them recovered but many were made worse. This was sad, not only for the patients and their families, but it was also a bitter disappointment for Koch who had up to then achieved so much success. His discovery of tuberculin however was not in vain, as its use in a certain test employed for the diagnosis of this condition subsequently proved of great value.

In 1904 he resigned from the Institute, and devoted the last six years of his life to travel and to the investigation of infectious diseases in the Tropics. Due to his development of appropriate methods most of the important micro-organisms had been thoroughly studied by the turn of the century and bacteriology had become a science in its own right.

Micro-organisms occur everywhere, and may be found in soil water and air, as well as in plants, animals and man. There are an enormous number of different types: most of them are harmless to man; some are helpful and are used in industry, as mentioned in the previous chapter, and only a few are harmful. They include protozoa, moulds, bacteria, higher bacteria, rickettsiales, mycoplasma, chlamydia and viruses.

Protozoa, usually regarded as the lowest form of animal life, are relatively large unicellular organisms whose protoplasm, unlike that of bacteria, is clearly differentiated into nucleus and cytoplasm. They may be saprophytes or parasites. Examples of protozoal parasites which affect man include those responsible for malaria and amoebic dysentery.

Moulds grow as branching filaments (hyphae) which interlace to form a meshwork (mycelium). They too may be saprophytic or parasitic, and in addition it is from species of two of these, known as

Penicillium and *Cephalosporium*, that the important antibacterial substances penicillin and the cephalosporins are obtained.

Bacteria are distinguished from unicellular plant life by not containing chlorophyll and not having demonstrable nuclei. They are divided into spherical cells known as cocci; cells in the shape of straight rods known as bacilli; also those in the shape of curved rods known as vibrios; in addition there are spiral flexible organisms known as spirochaetes. The last are structurally more complex than other bacteria and stain poorly with ordinary dyes; one of the most important spirochaetes is *Treponema pallidum*, the causative agent of syphilis.

Cocci and bacilli may be usefully divided into two main groups, namely Gram-positive and Gram-negative, based on a staining technique devised in 1884 by the Danish physician Hans Christian Joachim Gram (1853–1938). Gram published his famous staining method, which has since proved so useful in the classification of bacteria, whilst he was engaged in postgraduate studies in Germany at a time when Robert Koch and Koch's close friend and colleague Paul Ehrlich were popularizing the use of aniline dyes for staining bacteria in order to facilitate their examination under the microscope. Gram found that when he stained different types of bacteria with the aniline dye methyl violet followed by a solution of iodine, he could divide them into two groups according to whether the addition of alcohol resulted in the removal of the dye (Gram-negative group) or left it fixed to the cells (Gram-positive group).

Gram subsequently became a distinguished physician at the Royal Frederik's Hospital in Copenhagen and professor of pharmacology at the University there. He was greatly distressed by the uncritical use of many therapeutic substances at that time and did much to put pharmacology on a rational basis. He is mainly remembered however for his staining technique as this is in routine use in all bacteriological laboratories and because division of bacteria into his two groups has proved extremely useful in defining the range of activity of the various antibacterial substances which have become available during recent years.

Gram-positive cocci include staphylococci, streptococci and pneumococci. Staphylococci, which grow joined together in clusters

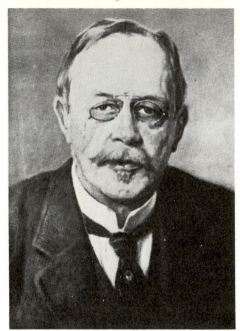

Fig. 17. Hans Christian Joachim Gram (1853–1938).

like bunches of grapes, are of two types; *Staphylococcus albus* a non-pathogen and *Staphylococcus aureus* a cause of serious disease in man.

Staphylococcus aureus is found living as a commensal* on normal skin and often in the nose of healthy people. In addition however it is one of the commonest causes of acute pyogenic (pus-producing) infection in man, including boils, carbuncles and abscesses, such as are found around the finger (whitlows) and in the lactating breast; also it is responsible for the disease in bone known as osteomyelitis, and in the lung is the cause of a highly infectious type of broncho-pneumonia. Further the organism may be responsible for food poisoning and is an important cause of sepsis in accidental wounds, surgical wounds and burns. Its spread into the blood stream is a not infrequent cause of a life-threatening septicaemia. Although many powerful anti-staphylococcal agents have been discovered during the

* From the Latin 'com' (together) and 'mensa' (table), i.e. an organism which sits with its host at table and shares the same food.

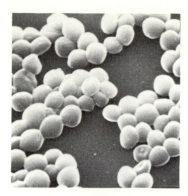 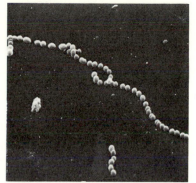

Fig. 18. An electron micrograph of Staphylococcus aureus *showing the characteristic 'bunch of grapes' formation.*

Fig. 19. An electron micrograph of Streptococcus pyogenes *showing the characteristic linear formation.*

past forty years, this organism continues to be a major threat to man's health for reasons that will be discussed in later chapters.

Streptococci take the form of spherical cells arranged in chains of varying length. There are three types including *Streptococcus viridans*, *S. faecalis*, and *S. pyogenes*. All of these are pathogenic to man but it is *Streptococcus pyogenes* which is responsible for over 90 per cent of human streptococcal infections, including tonsillitis, scarlet fever, erysipelas, cellulitis, and childbirth or puerperal fever. In addition it is a hypersensitivity reaction to *Streptococcus pyogenes* in the throat which is the cause of acute rheumatic fever and one form of acute nephritis. Healthy persons may be carriers of virulent streptococci in the throat.

Pneumococci are ovoid cells arranged in pairs. There are many types, with some of them growing as commensals in the nasopharynx of about 30 per cent of healthy people. These are capable of becoming pathogenic to their host once his resistance to infection is lowered for one reason or another. In addition there are others which are permanently virulent and capable of causing acute lobar pneumonia or meningitis in healthy people.

The Gram-negative cocci include gonococci and meningococci, both of which are found growing in pairs. The former is the cause of gonorrhoea and the latter of one type of meningitis.

The Gram-positive bacilli which are pathogenic to man include amongst others those responsible for anthrax, gas gangrene, tetanus, diphtheria, tuberculosis and leprosy. Anthrax causes widespread infection in animals, particularly sheep and cattle. The bacillus, which is a large, square-ended rod, is capable of survival in unfavourable conditions such as soil by the development of spores. The disease in man is mainly amongst those whose work brings them into contact either with animal skins, wool, hair or bristles. Important contributions to our understanding of this disease were made both by Robert Koch and by Louis Pasteur. Gas gangrene and tetanus are also caused by spore-bearing rods which grow freely in the soil. Gas gangrene is only likely to occur when there has been extensive damage to the tissues with contamination of a wound with soil such as occurs in war, road accidents and industrial injuries. Tetanus, commonly known as lockjaw from the intense spasm of the muscles of the face, is a much feared disease as it may result in widespread and very painful convulsive contractions of the muscles. This disease also occurs when wounds are contaminated with soil, particularly when this has been manured as the organism grows freely in the intestines of horses. In this disease the wound is often trivial such as that caused by a splinter, rusty nail or thorn prick.

Diphtheria, a disease caused by club-shaped bacilli, was at one time a dreaded life-threatening throat infection in children, but now in most developed countries is very rare due to effective immunization. Important pioneer work in the prevention both of tetanus and diphtheria was done in the closing years of the last century by von Behring, Kitasato and Paul Ehrlich.

The tubercle bacillus responsible for tuberculosis and the leprosy bacillus, although always included amongst Gram-positive organisms, are in fact very difficult to stain by Gram's technique. They are however readily stained by a method devised by Franz Ziehl and Adolf Neelsen in the last century, a technique which remains in routine use to this day.

The nomenclature employed in bacteriology has undergone a considerable change in recent years. Formerly the names given to bacteria were largely determined by morphological chacteristics, but as it is now realized that other properties also have to be taken into

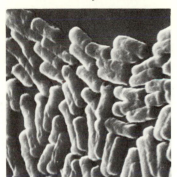

*Fig. 20. An electron micrograph
of* Escherichia coli.

account, they have all been renamed as part of an internationally
agreed scientific terminology. As however the general reader is likely
to be unfamiliar with and confused by many of these more recently
introduced names, they will for the most part be avoided. The story
told in these pages, for instance, will gain nothing by referring to the
tubercle bacillus as *Mycobacterium tuberculosis* or the gonococcus as
Neisseria gonorrhoeae. Nevertheless this does not apply in every case
and in referring to certain bacteria, especially the Gram-negative
bacilli, it is more expedient to use the international terminology.

Gram-negative bacilli may be divided into two main groups. One
group found in the intestine is collectively known as the Enterobacteriaceae and the other, because of the strikingly small size of the
organisms, is known collectively as the Parvobacteriaceae. The
Enterobacteriaceae include *Escherichia, Salmonella, Shigella, Klebsiella, Proteus*; and in addition there are the closely related *Pseudomonas*
and various vibrios.

Escherichia, named after Theodor Escherich, is the group of
bacteria which includes the very important *Escherichia coli* (formerly
known as *Bacterium coli*) and other coliform bacilli found in the
large intestine both in man and animals. These self-propelled, rod-
like organisms are present in everyone's gut, and are acquired during
the first few days of life by the child ingesting bacilli derived from its
mother or others in attendance. For the most part these organisms
are nothing more than harmless commensals but in recent years they

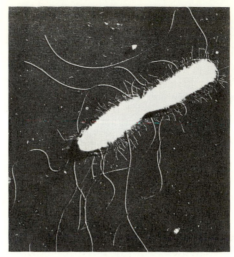

Fig. 21. An electron micrograph of Salmonella typhi, *the bacillus responsible for typhoid fever.*

have been found to be making an important contribution to the alarming spread of antibiotic resistance which is now occurring amongst various bacteria, a subject which will be discussed in detail in the final chapter. They are also a cause of acute enteritis in infants and on migrating from the gut are the cause of serious infection in the urinary and biliary tracts and of sepsis in surgical wounds and burns.

Salmonella, named after the American pathologist Daniel Elmer Salmon (1850–1940), is a group of self-propelled bacilli including the human pathogens *Salmonella typhi* and *S. paratyphi* A and B, the causes of typhoid and paratyphoid fever respectively. It also includes a large number of other organisms which although primarily animal pathogens are also capable of causing food poisoning in man, the commonest in Britain being *Salmonella typhimurium.*

Shigella, named after Kiyoshi Shiga, is a group of non-motile organisms responsible for the various types of bacillary dysentery. Some are highly virulent but fortunately *Shigella sonnei,* the one most often found in Britain, is the cause of a relatively mild disease. In both *Salmonella* and *Shigella* infections the source of organisms is faeces from a case or from a healthy carrier contaminating objects in the

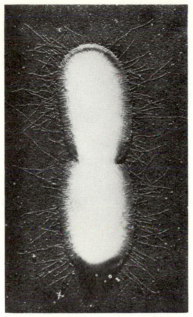

Fig. 22. An electron micrograph of Shigella flexneri. *One of a group of organisms responsible for bacillary dysentery.*

environment, especially food, either by direct contact or by flies acting as carriers.

Klebsiella, *Proteus* and *Pseudomonas* are free-living organisms widely distributed in soil and water. In addition they may at times be found as commensals in the intestinal tract. In recent years they have been assuming increasing importance as extremely dangerous pathogens in the urinary tract and in wounds and burns in patients confined within the closed environment of hospitals, due to the fact that the destruction of other bacteria more sensitive to the action of antibiotics has encouraged their proliferation.

The Parvobacteriaceae, a group of small, delicate Gram-negative rods includes amongst others *Pasteurella pestis*, the cause of plague, *Brucella abortus*, and *B. melitensis*, the causes of two types of undulant fever, and *Haemophilus** influenzae*, now the most important of them so far as this and certain other countries are concerned.

* From the Greek, 'haema' (blood), and 'pheilin' (to love).

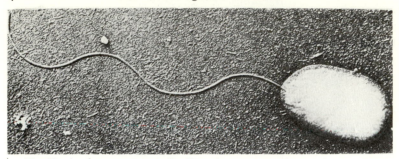

Fig. 23. An electron micrograph of Pseudomonas aeruginosa, *the organism formerly known as the* Pyocaneus bacillus (*p. 64*).

Haemophilus influenzae is a misnomer because although blood loving as the organism certainly is, growing readily on any culture material containing this substance, it is not the cause of influenza as was thought by Emil Pfeiffer when he gave it this name in 1892. He was led into this error by finding it in the sputum of those suffering from influenza in the pandemic which swept Europe during the preceding three years. Doubts about its causal relationship to influenza developed during and after the 1918–19 pandemic and of course were confirmed when in 1933 Smith, Andrewes and Laidlaw discovered the influenza virus. The organism is a very common commensal in the upper respiratory tract and an important pathogen together with the pneumococcus in acute exacerbations of infection in chronic bronchitis, a disease which causes such considerable morbidity and mortality, especially in Great Britain.

Higher bacteria, because they grow in in the form of branching filaments, have a certain resemblance to moulds. One important group, known as actinomycetes, live as parasites both in man and animals. Another group known as the streptomycetes is not pathogenic to man but they are widespread saprophytes in the soil and it is from these that so many antibiotics have been extracted during the past thirty years.

The rickettsiae and the chlamydiae are unicellular organisms with many of the characteristics of bacteria, but like viruses are incapable of living an independent existence, so that they are always found as parasites within the cells of a suitable host. The rickettsiae are found in lice, fleas and ticks and it is these which in turn are responsible for passing the organisms on to man with the production of various types of typhus fever, a disease which during the course of history has been an accompaniment of war, revolution and poverty.

The chlamydiae are widely distributed in birds and animals. Infected birds such as parrots, pigeons, hens, ducks, turkeys and canaries are capable of transmitting to man a severe form of broncho-pneumonia, known as psittacosis when parrots are responsible or otherwise ornithosis. A chlamydial organism is also responsible for trachoma, the commonest world-wide cause of blindness, with over five hundred million people infected particularly in the Middle East, India and China. In this country, as well as elsewhere, a similar organism is a parasite in the genital tract, causing in the male the common venereal disease known as non-specific urethritis and in women a symptomless cervicitis.

Mycoplasma are other very similar organisms occupying an intermediate position between bacteria and obligate intracellular organisms such as the rickettsiae and chlamydiae. This group includes the human pathogen *Mycoplasma pneumoniae*, a cause of one type of pneumonia.

Viruses, which are very much smaller than bacteria, can also grow and reproduce only in living cells. They are of many different kinds and are responsible for a very wide range of diseases, such as yellow fever, smallpox, chicken pox, mumps, measles, german measles, infective hepatitis, poliomyelitis, various types of encephalitis and meningitis, also some respiratory infections, influenza and even the more prosaic common or garden warts. Detailed consideration of these many viruses is outside the scope of this book, but of particular relevance in man's fight against bacteria is the special group of viruses known as bacteriophages or phages, which are parasites living and reproducing inside bacteria. A typical phage is tadpole-shaped with a polygonal 'head' consisting of deoxyribonucleic acid (DNA) surrounded by a thin protein membrane together with a short straight 'tail' which has a central hollow core. Phages attack bacteria by attaching themselves to the surface of bacterial cells by means of minute fibres at the tips of their 'tails' and then injecting their DNA into the cells. Once inside, the phage nucleic acid is reconstituted into so-called mature phages which eventually become

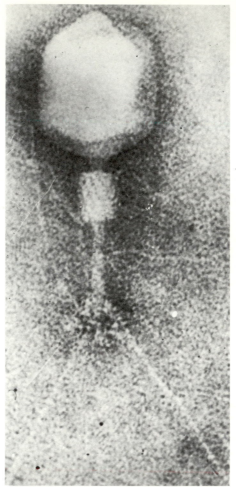

Fig. 24. Bacteriophage treated with hydrogen peroxide demonstrating the head filled with DNA, the tail, and the tail fibres.

so numerous as to cause the bacterial cell to burst. Man's many attempts over the years to make practical use of this destructive action of these viruses in the treatment of bacterial disease has so far proved unsuccessful, but paradoxically bacteria, and in particular staphylococci, at times derive much benefit from it. This is because, during

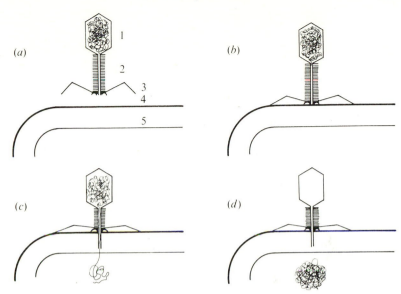

Fig. 25. Entry of bacteriophage DNA into a bacterial cell. (a) Free phage outside the cell with (1) head containing DNA, (2) tail with central core, (3) base plate with short spikes and fibres, (4) bacterial cell wall, and (5) cytoplasmic membrane. (b) Phage attaches to cell wall with fibres, base plate in close contact with outer layers of cell wall. (c) Tail contracts and central core is pushed through the cell wall and DNA transfer begins. (d) Transfer of DNA completed. Phage head is now empty and phage reproduction commencing in cell.

the process of intracellular phage reproduction the maturing viruses acquire a certain amount of the bacteria's DNA and in the case of some staphylococci this includes genetic information concerning bacterial resistance to antibiotics. Once the bacterial cell bursts and the phages are liberated, these in turn attack other staphylococci and during the course of this pass on to them this newly acquired genetic knowledge. Admittedly many of these bacteria die as a result of this aggressive action, but sufficient of them survive to make this method of transferring antibiotic resistance, technically known as 'transduction', a matter of serious consequence and one which therefore will be discussed again in the final chapter.

It was because bacteria form only a part of microscopic life that Sedillot, a surgeon, in 1878 introduced the term 'microbe' in the course of a discussion in the Paris Academy of Medicine, to describe any living organism so small as only to be visible under a microscope. The term has not become popular among scientists. Pasteur also considered that the term bacteriology was too limited and suggested that the science should be called microbiology.

Once micro-organisms could be identified, a search began for methods of combating those responsible for disease. This has not proved an easy task and progress when it has been made has often come when least expected and at times almost as if by chance.

It was not by chance, however, but through the pioneer work of Louis Pasteur, that the English surgeon Lister was able to develop a technique whereby the body could be opened and extensive operations performed without wounds becoming infected with bacteria from the surrounding air and from the hands and instruments of the surgeons. Hospital wards in his day were full of the stench of uncontrolled sepsis and patients' wounds dripped with pus, became gangrenous, and often gave rise to an overwhelming blood poisoning. Patients who came into hospital without much infection soon developed it once admitted and it was a frequent occurrence for the dreaded streptococcal infection called erysipelas to sweep through a hospital ward. The patients in those days had little chance to leave hospital alive; they might survive the hazards of extensive surgical procedures, but the possibility of withstanding attack by the countless bacteria present in the atmosphere of a hospital ward at that time was slight.

Joseph Lister, son of a London wine merchant, was professor of surgery in Edinburgh when he read how Louis Pasteur had shown that micro-organisms were responsible for the putrefaction of organic material and that different types of these bacteria were widely distributed in the atmosphere. He was much impressed by Pasteur's emphasis on the possible significance of this finding with regard to the spread of disease. Although Pasteur himself was not in a position to carry out experiments to prove it, Lister was convinced that infection in surgical wounds must be produced by germs from outside the body and searched for some chemical to destroy those found in the air, on surgical instruments and on surgeons' hands. He selected for his purpose carbolic acid which had first been prepared by a Manchester chemist named Calvert and which had already been used to

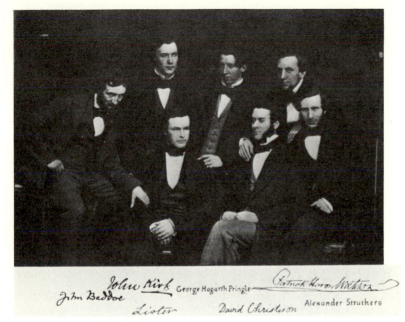

John Beddoe John Kirk George Hogarth Pringle Patrick Heron Watson
Lister David Christison Alexander Struthers

Fig. 26. Joseph Lister in 1854 at the age of twenty-seven with other young doctors at the Edinburgh Royal Infirmary.

deodorize and to disinfect sewage at Carlisle. He applied a dilute solution to all wounds and insisted that everything touching the wound, including the surgeons' hands, his instruments and dressings, must all be immersed in it.

Lister first used his antiseptic technique in March 1865, when he operated on a patient suffering from a compound fracture of the leg, and in 1867 published the results of treating such cases by this method. It was previously accepted that most patients with broken bones exposed to the air on account of extensive wounds, became seriously ill from infection, with the tissues covered in pus, so that it was often necessary to perform mutilating amputations, from which the patients frequently died. Lister however was able to report that out of eleven cases, who before this time would have certainly followed this course, nine recovered successfully, one had to undergo an amputation and only one died. This was a remarkable achievement and one of the most important landmarks in the history of

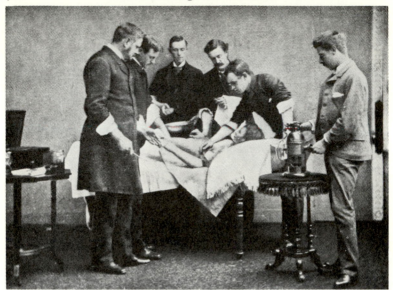

Fig. 27. A surgical operation at Aberdeen during the nineteenth century showing Lister's carbolic steam spray in use.

surgery. A year later he wrote a further article 'On the Antiseptic System of Treatment in Surgery'. He was fully conscious of his debt to Pasteur, who first inspired him to take up this work, and often publicly acknowledged this fact. In 1874 he wrote a letter to Pasteur in which he said 'Allow me to take this opportunity to tender you my most cordial thanks for having by your brilliant researches demonstrated to me the truth of the germ theory of putrefaction and thus furnished me with the principle upon which the antiseptic system could be carried out. Should you at any time visit Edinburgh, it would, I believe, give you sincere gratification to see at our hospital how largely mankind is being benefited by your labours.'

In spite of these outstanding results his ideas were not readily accepted and he had to face much criticism from sceptics both in this country and in other parts of the world. In 1877, he decided to give up his post of professor of surgery at Edinburgh, where he had been from 1869, to take an appointment at King's College Hospital, London. His Scottish students, unwilling to lose a successful and popular teacher, signed a petition asking him to reconsider his decision. He realized, however, that his method of antiseptic surgery was gaining acceptance and being applied daily in many parts of the world, but not in London, so he considered it was his duty to work there in order to show that surgery would never be safe until his technique was adopted. Thus he left his friends in Edinburgh, gave up a large private practice and started afresh at the age of fifty in a new and hostile environment. His London colleagues showed cold disinterest in his methods and openly snubbed him in front of students who in turn adopted an apathetic attitude and ignored him. Also the nurses, who had been working with eminent men of that day and who naturally enough had implicit faith in their methods, were rebellious and made no effort to hide their disapproval of his technique. But his results continued to be so outstanding that, after a short time, his critics were silenced and his method universally adopted. In recognition of his achievements he received the Order of Merit in 1902. He lived long enough to see how greatly his antiseptic method improved surgery all over the world before he died, in 1912, at the age of eighty-five. Many people wrote about his personality and his achievements but perhaps their sentiments were most aptly summed up in the report of the Royal College of Surgeons which said, 'His gentle nature, imperturbable temper, resolute will, indifference to ridicule and tolerance of hostile criticism, contrived to make him one of the noblest of men. His work will last for all time. Humanity will bless him for evermore and his fame will be immortal.'

4

DEFENCE MEASURES

It has long been recognized that there are certain diseases which, if survived, never attack the victim again. The Greek historian, Thucydides (464–404 B.C.), wrote that when plague was raging in Athens during the Peloponnesian wars the sick and dying would not have received attention had it not been for the devotion of those who had already suffered from it and who knew that they could not therefore catch it a second time. It was also well known in Ancient China that an adult, pock-marked from an attack of smallpox as a child, did not develop it again when exposed in an epidemic. It therefore soon became apparent that, once a person had overcome certain infections, a change took place in his body with the development of some defence mechanism which protected him from further attacks. Further, it was quickly recognized that this protective change inside the body could occur as a result of only a mild attack of the disease. The Chinese found that powder made from the dry crusts taken from a case of smallpox sniffed up the nose produced an attack of the disease, sufficiently mild not to be dangerous, but which at the same time gave protection from further attacks.

Smallpox was brought to Europe, from the Orient, by the Crusaders in the twelfth century. By the seventeenth century it had become widespread in Britain, with severe epidemics, in which one out of every four people infected died and many survivors were blinded and others grossly disfigured by the marks left by the pox. In 1717 Lady Mary Wortley Montagu, wife of the British Ambassador in Turkey, introduced inoculation into this country. The method used at that time was to induce a mild form of the disease, by drawing a thread, soaked in fluid from a smallpox pustule, through a small incision made into the arm. At first it was tried out on six condemned prisoners, and after it had been shown to be successful with them, several members of the royal household were inoculated. Following this, it became an established practice, and people clamoured to have

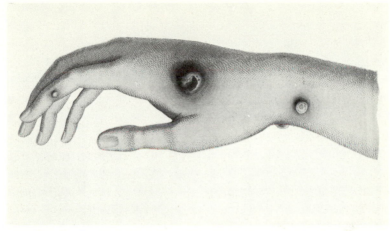

Fig. 28. The hand of a milkmaid, Sarah Nelmes, infected with cowpox from which Jenner conceived the idea of vaccination.

the disease artificially induced. The Quaker physician, Thomas Dimsdale (1712–1800), practised it widely, and became so famous that news of him reached the Empress Catherine of Russia who summoned him to St Petersburg to inoculate herself and her son. He was fearful lest something might go wrong and planned how he would escape should any disaster occur; he must have felt very relieved when he was able to write in his diary 'She has had the smallpox in the most desirable manner which now thank God is over!' He had good cause for anxiety because the disease produced in this way although usually mild was not always so; also, it was as contagious as the naturally occurring disease and required the isolation of the patient for a number of weeks.

As there were these serious disadvantages, people were only too willing to abandon this method of immunization as soon as a better one was found. It had been a popular belief for some time amongst country folk that a person infected from cows with a mild variety of pox was protected from the far more serious condition of smallpox. This was brought to the notice of the Gloucestershire medical practitioner, Edward Jenner (1749–1823), when he diagnosed smallpox in a dairymaid, who immediately told him that this was impossible as she had already suffered from cowpox. He decided to make some

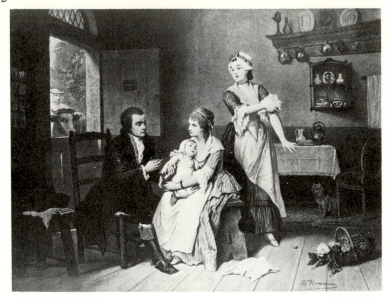

Fig. 29. Edward Jenner vaccinating a child with fluid taken from a blister on the hand of Sarah Nelmes who had contracted cowpox whilst milking.

observations about this for himself and closely studied the effect of smallpox inoculation in patients already known to have had cowpox. He found that the reaction around the incision, in such patients, was negligible and there was no general constitutional disturbance. This convinced him that the dairymaid was right about cowpox giving protection against smallpox. In May 1796 he induced cowpox in an eight-year-old boy by the insertion of some fluid into his arm, obtained from blisters on the hand of a young woman suffering from this disease. Next, he inoculated him with fluid taken from a case of smallpox and no reaction occurred. Thus, for the first time, a person had been protected from smallpox by the artificial introduction of the milder form of pox which normally affects cows. It was for this reason that this preventive technique became known as vaccination, from the Latin word *vacca*—a cow.

As with all new and revolutionary ideas, there was much criticism and scepticism about the method, so that Jenner received strong opposition from many of his colleagues, particularly as, at that time, it was not free from complications. Occasionally, it led to bad ulcers

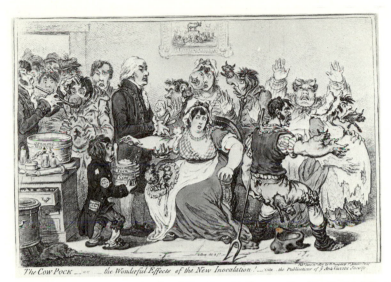

The Cow Pock_or_ the Wonderful Effects of the New Inoculation !_

Fig. 30. A cartoon on vaccination 'The Cow Pock—or—the Wonderful Effects of the New Inoculation' by Gillray, spokesman for many fierce opponents of vaccination.

developing at the site of inoculation and, in addition, some patients developed smallpox in spite of having been vaccinated. Nevertheless, it was soon realized that the benefits far outweighed any of these disadvantages and the method was widely practised. Jenner became famous and his country rewarded him for his outstanding contribution to medical science by a parliamentary grant of £10,000 in 1802 and a further £20,000 in 1806.

Knowledge of his technique soon spread abroad, and the success of vaccination against smallpox encouraged people to develop similar methods of preventive inoculation against other diseases prevalent at that time. A Frenchman, Auzias-Turenne, believed that it might be possible to prevent the ravages of syphilis by inoculation with a mild form of the disease and went so far as to advocate to the Paris Academy of Medicine that this should be performed on all the youth of France! He also believed that it would prove possible to develop methods to protect people against other diseases, such as anthrax, cholera and rabies; although he himself was not able to achieve this, he attained a good theoretical understanding of the subject, as is shown in his book entitled *La Syphilisation*, published in 1878. It is obvious that his ideas were closely studied by medical research workers at that time, and it is said that Louis Pasteur, who had developed a particular interest in this subject as a result of being much impressed by Jenner's work on smallpox vaccination, often read and made copious notes from the book, determined to find similar methods to apply to other diseases. An accident which occurred about a year after the book was published gave Pasteur his first important lead. In the spring of 1879 he began to study cholera in chickens. Towards the end of the summer, he took some chicken cholera bacteria from an old culture which had been in the laboratory for some months and injected them into healthy chickens, in the hope of inducing the disease. He was not successful. Therefore, he obtained a fresh supply of bacteria, from chickens already suffering from the disease, and when these were injected into healthy chickens, they readily induced the illness. Next, he injected these virulent organisms into chickens which had already been given bacteria from the old culture and once again he failed to produce any ill effects. Pasteur, with his great ability for accurate deduction, realized what must have happened. The chicken cholera bacteria kept in his laboratory all through the summer had lost most of their virulence and power to produce disease but, when injected into chickens, they still had the ability to bring about changes which made the chickens immune to further attack by virulent organisms. He had thus stumbled upon another disease against which artificial immunity could be induced. In order to show that the process was somewhat akin to Jenner's use of cowpox, he referred to this also as vaccination and the term has subsequently been used for many other types of immunization. This observation with chickens was of fundamental importance as it led him and others to work out similar methods of vaccination against other infections, so that today there are highly effective methods of immunization against a wide variety of diseases.

He discovered that to make disease-producing bacteria lose their virulence it was necessary to employ a different technique in each case. Within four years he had been successful with four conditions, of which two, anthrax and rabies, affect man. He studied anthrax because of observations he made on sheep affected with this disease.

He had noticed that a flock of sheep grazing for a long time in a field where an animal which had died of anthrax had been buried, were not harmed when virulent anthrax bacilli were injected into them, whereas a similar injection into other sheep resulted in death. He deduced from this that the healthy sheep must have absorbed small amounts of anthrax bacteria from the dead animal and that this had brought about protective changes in their bodies, with the production of resistance to the disease. He therefore devised a method of growing anthrax bacteria in the laboratory by which they lost most of their virulence, and found that these attenuated organisms, on injection into animals, protected them from the effects of virulent bacteria. This was a very important observation because anthrax was prevalent in animals at that time and the cause of much financial loss to farmers. Many people however would not accept Pasteur's claims and his enemies, at the instigation of a veterinary surgeon named Rossignol, set out to ridicule him by staging a large-scale, much publicized experiment. Animals were taken to Rossignol's fields at Pouilly le Fort, near Melun, and a number vaccinated with Pasteur's attenuated bacilli and then inoculated some days later with virulent germs; at the same time, as a control, a similar number were inoculated with virulent germs alone. The vaccinated animals consisted of twenty-four sheep, one goat and six cows, and the controls consisted of twenty-four sheep, one goat and four cows. On 2 June 1881 a great crowd assembled to watch the result of the experiment. Pasteur approached the farm somewhat nervously, only to find however on arrival that all cynicism had disappeared and that everyone there was full of admiration and respect for him; the experiment had fully justified his claims. All the vaccinated sheep and cows were well; twenty-one of the control sheep were dead, two others died that morning in front of the crowd and the last one died at the end of the day. Also, the four control cows were ill. Obviously, with results like these, it was not long before anthrax immunization was widely practised with an enormous reduction in the death-rate amongst sheep.

A few months after his triumph at Pouilly le Fort, Pasteur attended the Medical Congress in London, where he suggested that when referring to the various methods of immunization which were being discovered the terms 'vaccine' and 'vaccination' should be used in all cases, in order to pay tribute to 'the merit and immense services rendered by one of the greatest men of England, your Jenner'.

Pasteur's interest in anthrax immunization obviously arose because his initial observations with sheep had suggested to him that immunization to this disease might be a possibility, and because the disease was widespread and affecting the nation's economy. His reason for wishing to develop a method of immunization against rabies was rather less obvious as it was not a disease which caused many deaths by comparison with other far more prevalent diseases, the causative germ had not been identified and, since it chiefly affected dogs and wolves, experiments were difficult and costly. It is, however, an extremely distressing and fatal disease which can affect anyone attacked by an infected animal. The other name for it, hydrophobia, literally translated means fear of water, because of the alarming convulsions a patient undergoes at the sight of water. These may be induced by offering the person a glass of water. As the glass touches the mouth, the head is thrown back in a series of spasmodic jerks, breathing becomes difficult and any water reaching the mouth is immediately ejected. These violent convulsions are brought about by painful spasms in the muscles which control swallowing and breathing and make the disease intensely frightening both for the sufferer and onlookers. It is said that Pasteur's interest in rabies was stimulated by vivid memories of the time when, during his childhood, an infected wolf attacked a number of men in his village. He watched while one of the victims had his bites cauterized with a red hot iron at a blacksmith's shop, in an attempt to prevent the development of the disease and later he learnt that many of them died after prolonged suffering.

As Pasteur knew that the causative organisms of rabies attacked the brain and spinal cord, he took spinal cords from rabbits which had died from the disease and suspended the cords in dry sterile air. He found that, as a result of this process, the rabies organisms in the nervous tissue lost their virulence and he could then use an emulsion of these cords as a vaccine. This vaccine was first used in dogs, was found to be effective and later saved many people from suffering. At first he had to face much bitter opposition and criticism from

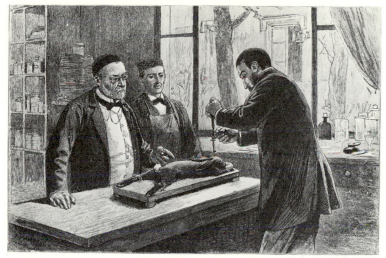

Fig. 31. *Louis Pasteur watching as the spinal cord from a rabbit killed by rabies is removed for use in preparing vaccine against this disease.*

colleagues, who considered the method to be highly dangerous, but ultimately the discovery was to make him famous.

A person bitten by a rabid dog does not necessarily contract the disease; it depends on the number and character of the bites and on which part of the body they are inflicted. For the disease to develop, the germs have to travel from the bite to invade the central nervous system, and the time which elapses between the person being bitten and the development of symptoms is usually about one or two months. Pasteur suggested that advantage might be taken of this long interval, by vaccinating a person soon after he had been bitten, so that some immunity could be developed by the time the organism reached the brain and spinal cord. He carried out experiments by inoculating dogs bitten by rabid animals and the results appeared to be promising. It needed much courage however to take the next step and to inject the vaccine into a human being exposed to the disease for, not only might the patient not develop symptoms if left untreated, there was also a chance that the vaccine itself might cause trouble. Pasteur was therefore very hesitant about using it, especially as well-informed medical opinion considered it to be an unwarranted risk, but he was forced to act when Joseph Meister, a boy aged nine, was

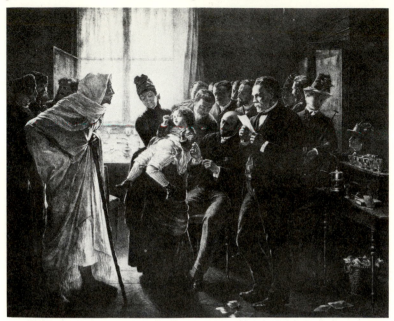

Fig. 32. Louis Pasteur watching a child being immunized against rabies.

brought to him from Alsace on 6 July 1885 suffering from bites on the hands, legs and thighs, from a rabid dog. Pasteur knew that the chances of the boy getting rabies from the bites were very high and felt he could not just stand by to watch this happen, so he gave him a course of injections, which to his great relief had no ill effects. The boy returned safely to Alsace. When this lad grew up he became a gatekeeper at the Pasteur Institute in Paris, where he died in 1940, for rather than let the German invaders force him to open the crypt where Pasteur was buried, he committed suicide.

The second case treated by Pasteur was that of Jean Baptiste Jupille, a fifteen-year-old shepherd, who saw a dog about to savage some children. He attacked it with his whip, but in so doing received numerous extensive bites. The dog was subsequently found to be suffering from rabies and the boy was rushed to Paris for treatment. He fortunately survived and his great bravery towards those children is commemorated in a statue which stands today in front of the Pasteur Institute.

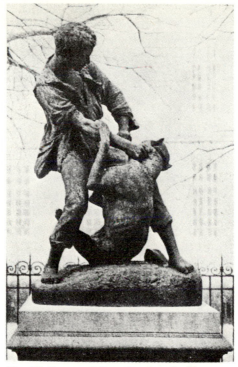

Fig. 33. Statue of Jean Baptiste Jupille, commemorating Pasteur's second case of treatment of rabies and Jupille's act of bravery in protecting children.

These two dramatic recoveries were soon widely reported, so that before long, a large number of people bitten by dogs demanded vaccination from Pasteur. This method of treatment was much criticized by his colleagues, who argued that few people who are bitten develop the disease, and that the vaccine itself was equally dangerous. He had a certain number of failures, which were made much of by his opponents, but an English Commission, set up in 1888, to investigate the validity of his claims, expressed confidence in the value of his work in the following words: 'From the evidence of all these facts we think it is certain that the inoculations practised by M. Pasteur on persons bitten by rabid animals have prevented the occurrence of hydrophobia in a large proportion of those who, if they had not been so inoculated, would have died of the disease.' The Commission also recognized that by this technique he had established a new method which might be applicable against other diseases. 'We believe that the value of this discovery will be found much greater than can be estimated by its present utility for it shows that it may become possible to avert by inoculation even after infection other diseases besides hydrophobia.'

This was the real crux of the matter, for, although immunization against rabies may not have been more successful in reducing the number of deaths from the disease than have strict laws enforcing the muzzling of dogs, it was his work on rabies, anthrax and other diseases that established important basic principles. It showed that it is possible to reduce the virulence of organisms, so that, when injected into animals or man in this weakened state, they do not cause harm, but set up protective changes. Since that time, it has been possible to apply this to other diseases, including diphtheria, whooping cough, typhoid fever, tetanus, tuberculosis, yellow fever and, more recently, poliomyelitis.

5

THE ENEMY UNDER ATTACK

The earlier chapters have shown that in the struggle against disease it was only possible to adopt commonsense general rules of hygiene until, with the discovery of the microscope, the enemy was identified. It was then possible to develop more accurate defence measures, including a technique to prevent the introduction of infection into wounds during surgical operations, and the stimulation of the natural defence mechanisms of the body by vaccination. The next step in the war against disease-producing bacteria would be to kill them in a direct manner with some chemical poison, but it was soon realized that this would present difficulties, as any poison which would kill bacteria was just as likely to damage the tissue cells of the body. A certain amount of encouragement, however, was derived from the fact that, during the course of centuries, a few chemical substances had accidentally been found to be effective against a small number of diseases.

As long ago as the sixteenth century the use of the metal antimony was advocated by that colourful character Paracelsus (1493–1541) whose real name, in keeping with his flamboyant personality, was Philippus Theophrastus Aureolus Bombastus von Hohenheim. He styled himself Paracelsus because, with his singular lack of humility, he wished to be identified with Celsus, the celebrated Roman medical author, whose eight famous books, entitled *De re Medicina*, were written about A.D. 30. Paracelsus has been accused of many hard things: charlatanism, drunkenness and boastfulness; some said he was mad. Nevertheless, he was a prolific and provocative writer. One famous book which is now acknowledged to have been written by him had the somewhat strange title *The Triumphal Chariot of Antimony* (1604); in this, he recommended the medicament for a wide variety of maladies without offering much evidence upon which to base his faith in its efficacy. Since that time however it has proved to be of great value in the treatment of many tropical infections.

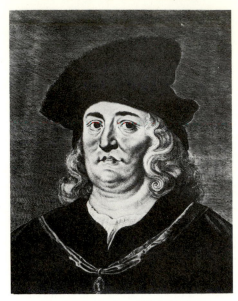

Fig. 34. Paracelsus (1493–1541).

Paracelsus is also said to have introduced mercury in the treatment of syphilis; this was certainly sound practice, as time has confirmed its value in this disease and, in fact, it continued to be used long after certain arsenical compounds were discovered by Ehrlich at the beginning of this century.

Another microbial disease which has been successfully treated with a chemical substance for several centuries is malaria, the cause of much suffering and death in many parts of the world. A specific cure for it, introduced to Europe in the seventeenth century, was found in the bark of the cinchona tree which grows in South America. In Great Britain its use against malaria, a serious and prevalent disease at that time, was popularized by the famous physician Thomas Sydenham (1624–89). For a long time there was a romantic legend that cinchona bark was first brought to Europe by Lady Ana de Osorino, Countess of Chinchon, the wife of the Viceroy of Peru. It was said that when she was in Lima, early in the seventeenth century, she developed malaria, and at the suggestion of a local governor, took some powder prepared from the bark of the tree, and was miraculously cured. In gratitude for this, she distributed large quantities of the powder to the citizens of Lima, and later introduced it into Spain. Unfortunately the story is not true, because A. W. Haggis, writing in the *Bulletin of the History of Medicine* in 1941, states that he has studied the diary of the Countess and found that she died in Spain before her husband was ever sent to Peru, and that his second wife, who did go to Peru with him, not only was never ill there, but died on the return journey before she reached home. It would seem that the truth is that the bark was introduced into Europe from South America by Jesuit missionaries and priests.

At the beginning of the nineteenth century, the German Sertürner, extracted morphine from opium in poppies. This stimulated two young French chemists, Pelletier and Caventou, to attempt to separate active ingredients from other plants. From a South American plant, called ipecacuanha, they extracted emetine which has since been found to have a specific action against the parasite responsible for amoebic dysentery. Later, by a similar method, they separated the active principles in cinchona bark and, when they reported this discovery in 1820, called the part which cured malaria quinine, a name derived from the old Peruvian word for the cinchona tree, quina-quina.

About this time, on account of the world demand for this drug, which only came from trees in South America, certain nations with Eastern dependencies where malaria was rife, particularly the British and the Dutch, became alarmed in case the supply should be insufficient for their needs. The British therefore transferred seeds and plants to India and Ceylon, and the Dutch to Java. At first the British seemed to be more successful, as their plantations in India grew hardy trees (*Cinchona succi rubra*) but it was found that this particular species gave a poor yield of quinine. The Dutch, on the other hand, had the good fortune to buy, by chance, a small quantity of seeds from an Englishman, Charles Ledger, who had lived in Peru for a long time; it turned out that the trees from these seeds (later called *Cinchona ledgerina*) gave an exceptionally high yield of quinine, but unfortunately proved very difficult to rear. The Dutch overcame this difficulty by grafting them on to robust trees of the *Cinchona succi rubra* variety, and by this means established trees in

Java, as hardy as the British ones in India, but giving a very much greater yield of quinine.

Mercury against syphilis and quinine against malaria were therefore two of the earliest examples of chemical substances which, when taken into the body, killed disease-producing micro-organisms. They were first used long before the specific micro-organisms had been identified, as it was not until 1880 that Alphonse Laveran, a young medical officer in the French army stationed in Algeria, first demonstrated the malarial parasite in the red cells of patients, nor until 1905, that Fritz Schaudinn, in Germany, identified the organism responsible for syphilis.

The identification of bacteria under the microscope towards the end of the last century stimulated the German chemist, Paul Ehrlich, to search systematically for chemical substances which, when taken into the body, would kill harmful bacteria, while doing as little damage as possible to the tissue cells. It was about this time that aniline dyes were first manufactured and found to be not only of great value in the textile industry but also in the newly developed science of microscopy, as they stained tissue cells and bacterial cells vivid colours, thus allowing a detailed examination of them to be made under the microscope. It was noticed that these dyes were absorbed by different types of cells in a highly selective manner so that each type stood out in its own distinctive colour. This observation led Ehrlich to consider whether he could find a dye which would specifically adhere to bacteria in the body, and thus kill them, but which, at the same time, would not affect other cells. The development of this idea led him eventually to discover important antibacterial drugs, and, by the adoption of a similar approach, his pupil, Gerard Domagk, discovered further ones of great value after the First World War.

Paul Ehrlich was the first man to place the search for antibacterial chemical substances on a scientific basis and it was he who introduced the term 'chemotherapy' for this type of treatment, the use of which has now been extended to include the killing of cancer cells by similar substances.

It is a commonplace observation that certain animals help man by killing others that may be harmful to him but it is less well known that this also occurs in life visible only through the microscope. This phenomenon is readily demonstrated by a study of the micro-organisms in the soil. Animals excrete a large number of bacteria into the soil and infected animals are also buried there but, in spite of this, it is not the source of much disease. This is because organisms deposited in it are quickly killed, partly by the action of the sun, but also by other microbes which live there. It was an appreciation of this which led Selman Waksman to discover streptomycin. In addressing the National Academy of Sciences in Washington, in 1940, he said 'Bacteria pathogenic for man and animals find their way to the soil, either in the excreta of the hosts or in their remains. If one considers the period for which animals and plants have existed on this planet and the great number of disease-producing microbes that must have thus gained entrance into the soil, one can only wonder that the soil harbours so few bacteria capable of causing infectious diseases in man and in animals. The soil was searched for bacterial agents of infectious diseases until the conclusion was reached that these do not survive long in the soil. The cause of the disappearance of these disease-producing organisms in the soil is to be looked for among the soil-inhabiting microbes antagonistic to the pathogens and bringing about their rapid destruction in the soil.'

This observation suggested to him that it might be possible to use some of these microbes which kill bacteria in the soil, or suitable extracts from them, to kill bacteria causing diseases in the body. This proved highly successful and many important antibiotics derived from soil microbes, in addition to streptomycin, have been produced.

The word antibiosis was first used, in 1889, by the Frenchman, Vuillemin, who said 'when two living bodies are closely united and one of the two exercises a destructive action on a more or less extensive portion of the other then we can say that "antibiosis" exists'. After this its use was mainly confined to the activities of micro-organisms, but the term antibiotic was originally an adjective applied to any organism which had a lethal effect on other organisms. Its modern usage as a noun, when referring to substances such as penicillin and streptomycin, began in 1941, when Waksman employed it to describe any chemical substance extracted from a micro-organism which had the ability to kill other pathogenic microbes.

Although much progress in the conquest of disease has been achieved during this century by the skilful utilization of the lethal effects of certain microbes on others, it should be made clear that the possibility was first considered as long ago as 1877. At that time Louis Pasteur, with his colleague Joubert, observed that anthrax bacilli growing in urine were often killed when the specimen became contaminated by other organisms from the air. They also noticed that animals infected with anthrax bacilli often did not die from this disease if, at the same time, they were also infected by other organisms. These observations led Pasteur to prophesy that, 'the time may come when we may utilise harmless microbes for combating harmful ones'.

Cantani, in 1885, had the original and ingenious idea, based on this principle that micro-organisms might be used to attack harmful bacteria in the lungs. He attempted this by trying to kill the bacilli causing pulmonary tuberculosis in a patient, by insufflating into the lungs large quantities of ill-defined harmless organisms. This was the first time micro-organisms had been introduced into a patient's body in an effort to kill disease-producing bacteria.

In the laboratory similar efforts were made to inhibit the growth of organisms on culture plates by the action of others. A Swiss, Garré, in 1887 published work on this and in 1904 W. D. Frost, in Great Britain, described several methods for investigating the antagonistic properties of bacteria. Frost grew one type of bacteria in a liquid medium in a flask and another in a medium contained in a collodion sac suspended in the flask. He found that a substance which today would be called an antibiotic, produced by the bacteria in one medium, could diffuse through the collodion membrane and inhibit the growth of bacteria in the other.

In 1887, Emmerich, in Germany, showed that some protection could be given to rabbits suffering from experimental anthrax by the simultaneous injections of streptococci and in 1889, Bouchard, in France, reported that rabbits infected with this disease could be helped by the injection of organisms called pyocyaneus bacilli. Following this Emmerich and Low, ten years later, prepared an extract from these organisms called pyocyanase and found that, in the laboratory, this was capable of killing anthrax bacilli, typhoid bacilli, diphtheria bacilli, staphylococci and the causative organisms of plague. Therefore, they attempted to inject it into experimentally infected animals, but it proved too toxic and could only be used by local application. Thus, by the turn of the century, many attempts had been made to apply the principle of antibiosis and the successful extraction of pyocyanase gave promise that it might be possible to find similar, but more suitable, antibiotics in the future.

When Waksman began his search for antibiotic substances, in 1939, the first organism which he studied was once again the pyocyaneus bacillus, and its extract pyocyanase. Although pyocyanase, as before, did not prove very suitable as an antibiotic, its preparation helped him to develop a suitable technique for the extraction and purification of other substances from micro-organisms and allowed him to establish satisfactory methods for testing their properties.

Microbes which he next investigated included the actinomycetes, organisms at one time known as 'ray fungi' from their appearance under the microscope, and the closely related streptomycetes. It was from a species of the latter that in 1943 he obtained streptomycin, the drug which was to play such a vital part in the control of tuberculosis, in addition to being useful against other infections.

He was not the first to work with actinomycetes. Much evidence had been produced long before this to show that these organisms, and extracts from them, had the power to kill other microbes. In 1917 Greig-Smith, in Australia, reported that he had noted that actinomycetes recovered from the soil had the power of stopping the growth of certain bacteria. Lieske, in 1921, published a monograph in German on *The Morphology and Biology of the Ray Fungi*, in which he discussed antibacterial chemical substances produced by the actinomycetes. Work on the same subject was published in French medical journals, by Gratia and Dath, in 1924 and 1925, and again by Gratia in 1934.

Similarly, Alexander Fleming's observations on the adverse effect of a mould on the growth of some staphylococci in 1928, which led to the discovery of penicillin, was not the first occasion on which a mould had been observed to have antibacterial properties. As long ago as 1896 Gosio described how he had obtained a crystalline substance from a mould of the penicillium family, which inhibited the growth of anthrax bacilli, and regretted that he was unable to perform animal experiments because of lack of material. Also, in 1913,

Vaudremer published in a French medical journal an account of the effect of another mould, the *Aspergillus fumigatus*, which he found 'digested' the tubercle bacillus. As a result of this he carried out animal experiments, and injected filtrates of the mould into patients suffering from tuberculosis.

It may therefore be seen that the progress made in the twentieth century had its roots in the past. Further, it has to be realized that, even when this progress was made, final victory was not achieved easily, or quickly, but was dependent on the contributions of a large number of workers. For example, from the time that Fleming first made his original observation on the effect of a mould (subsequently identified as *Penicillium notatum*), it was another ten years before it achieved practical importance, when Florey, Chain and their team of workers at Oxford developed a technique which allowed them to produce an extract which was suitably purified for clinical use. Repeated attempts by various chemists before this had failed and it looked, at one time, as if the task might not be possible.

This chapter has outlined the evolution of ideas which led eventually to the discovery of important drugs for the treatment of microbial disease during this century. These discoveries had to wait until there were appropriate economic and social stimuli and until suitable progress has been made in the development of the ancillary sciences, but they could never have been achieved without the initial inspiration of pioneers. René Dubos in his book *Louis Pasteur* has a chapter devoted to the 'Mechanisms of Discovery' in which he says, 'because every discovery, even that which appears to first sight the most original and intuitive can always be shown to have roots deep in the past, certain students of the history of science believe that the role of the individual in the advancement of knowledge is in reality very small'. It is certainly true that any great discovery which is made by a research worker often depends on the valuable work of others in the past as well as on the good fortune that he is working on a given problem at the right time in the right place. When therefore we praise the men who have made great discoveries we should also remember all the other workers, sometimes nameless and often long forgotten, who prepared the way. In the next chapters the discovery of present-day antibacterial drugs will be discussed, beginning with the work of Paul Ehrlich, the father of modern chemotherapy.

6

GUIDED MISSILES

Paul Ehrlich, the only son of an inn-keeper, was born at Strehlen, Upper Silesia, in March 1854. His grandfather had been a keen scientist and Paul resembled him in appearance and aptitude. His father was not a practical man and the successful running of their business was due to his mother's drive and ability. Paul showed his interest in chemistry at an early age so that by the time he was eight the chemists in his town were already making cough drops according to his prescription! At school he was always trying out new chemical experiments. Latin and mathematics pleased him but he found German composition to be extremely difficult. His inability to write a competent essay nearly failed him in his school-leaving examinations; fortunately he had done well enough in his other subjects to compensate for this weakness.

After leaving school, he went to Breslau University but was unhappy there and moved during his first term to the newly founded University of Strasbourg. He was fortunate in Strasbourg to be taught by Professor Waldeyer, an outstanding chemist, who took a great interest in young Ehrlich, and encouraged him to do original work while only a student. His main interest right from the start was in the new aniline dyes which were then being produced in a German chemical works and, on his own initiative, he explored various ways in which these could be used to stain cells so as to make it easier to study them under the microscope. He was to continue this study throughout his time at the university and was responsible for the development of techniques which made a considerable contribution to the science of microscopy. He did not allow it however to interfere with his other studies, and in his third term at the university passed his 'Physikum'—an examination which is held at German universities in chemistry, botany, zoology, physics, anatomy and physiology. After this, he continued his medical studies by returning to the university at Breslau. One day a physician from the town of

Wollstein in Silesia visited the university to show the professor his work on the anthrax bacillus. He was conducted through the various laboratories and while there saw a student working industriously at his bench, 'That is little Ehrlich, who is very good at staining but will never pass his examinations', he was told. This was the first introduction that the famous bacteriologist, Robert Koch, had to the student who was not only to pass his examinations but, in later years, was to work in close collaboration with him.

He completed his university training at Leipzig where he continued his studies with dyes, not only in the laboratory but also in the little inn where he lodged. Years later, when he became famous, the inn-keeper's daughter wrote to him to remind him of the time when all the towels in the house were marked with dyes in every shade of red and blue. Even the billiard table itself had suffered in the same way, for he made his experiments on this as there was nowhere else suitable.

It was at Leipzig, in the year 1878, that he graduated at the age of twenty-four as a doctor of medicine. His thesis for this degree dealt with the use of aniline dyes to stain preparations of tissue cells so that they might be studied under the microscope. In this thesis, he clearly brought out the basic principle that every dye has an affinity for certain specific types of cell, so that the one becomes readily bound to the protoplasm of the other. This fundamental observation later led him to examine the dyes again in a search for chemicals which might kill the cells of bacteria in the body, whilst leaving the surrounding tissue cells unaffected. It will thus be seen that this initial work of Ehrlich's, done before he was qualified as a doctor, served as the guide which led him to create the science of chemotherapy.

It is somewhat alarming to discover that, with the passing of years, this important thesis became lost in the archives of the university at Leipzig and it was only after his death that his wife and his friend Professor Leonor Michaelis succeeded in tracing the original. He actually published the main theme of his dissertation in a journal in 1877, one year before his thesis was presented to the university. Miss Martha Marquardt, his secretary from 1902 until the time of his death, has in recent years found a copy of this journal in the British Museum.

After qualifying as a doctor, Ehrlich became a house physician to Professor von Frerichs at the Charité Hospital in Berlin. The Professor immediately recognized the great ability of this young man and encouraged him in his research work. Ehrlich continued to take a special interest in the application of dyes and developed methods of staining samples of blood so that the various cells in it could readily be identified under the microscope. He was the first man to show that the white cells could be separated by their staining reactions into three distinct types; an observation which has proved of great practical importance. He soon became famous for this alone and professors from other universities travelled far to watch him demonstrate his methods. They were not only very impressed by his skill, but amazed by the simplicity of his apparatus, which consisted of nothing more than an iron plate on a tripod over a gas jet, some slides and a few dyes.

While he was still a house physician, he married the nineteen-year-old daughter of an industrialist in Upper Silesia. She was to remain his devoted and understanding companion for the rest of his life. There must have been times when she wished she saw more of him, because like many great men, he became heavily committed with his work and so devoted to his research studies that it was difficult to persuade him to take even a short holiday. He drove himself hard and rarely stopped to take proper meals but seemed to exist by drinking large quantities of mineral waters and smoking countless cigars. His energy was boundless and he fired all those around him with similar enthusiasm. He would always find time to explain his theories to anyone who was interested and would illustrate these theories by drawing with chalk on furniture, doors, or even the listener himself. His words would be punctuated by the frequent use of characteristic interjections which later in life became almost proverbial. One of his favourite expressions was, 'You see: you understand.' This frequent interjection also figured in his dictation, so that his first secretary at times became so confused that she included it in the typescript, to produce very curiously worded documents. Finally, the effort of concentrating to take down only the essentials proved too much and she found herself quite unable to do the work and ran away.

In 1882 Ehrlich attended a meeting of the Physiological Society of

Berlin when Robert Koch announced his momentous discovery of the tubercle bacillus. Immediately the lecture was finished, Ehrlich rushed back to his laboratory at the Charité Hospital, to stain with dyes, specimens of sputum coughed up by tuberculous patients. As it was late at night he looked round hastily for somewhere to put the slides to dry: he noticed the iron stove was cold, as the fire had been out for some hours, so he quickly put the slides down on the top of this. The next morning when the cleaner arrived, she lit the fire as usual not noticing the slides. Ehrlich arrived soon after to examine his specimens and to his horror saw what had happened. He rushed forward in dismay and quickly snatched them up, but to his amazement, after suitable treatment he found that they were successfully stained and on examining them under a microscope, the tubercle bacilli were seen to stand out very clearly as masses of short red sticks heaped together in clumps. By this lucky accident, he stumbled upon the important truth that staining of tubercle bacilli is best accomplished by heating the dye.

Ehrlich immediately informed Koch of his discovery and this was the beginning of a friendship and successful partnership in various research projects. Koch paid tribute to the importance of Ehrlich's work on the staining of tubercle bacilli in an article published in 1883, in which he said, 'It was soon found that, with Ehrlich's method of staining, the recognition of tubercle bacilli could readily be made use of in diagnosis'.

Life was going smoothly for Ehrlich when his chief, Professor von Frerichs, suddenly died. Unfortunately his successor, Professor Gerhardt, and Ehrlich found themselves to be at cross purposes and the friendly happy atmosphere changed to one where there was persistent tension. His new chief demanded that he should carry out dull routine clinical duties and discouraged him from doing any original work. Ehrlich, who had a sensitive personality, felt his spirit to be crushed and through frustration, became physically and mentally exhausted. To add to his troubles, before long, he began to show signs that he had developed pulmonary tuberculosis. He therefore resigned his post at the hospital and with his wife, went to live in Egypt for a time. It would seem that his tuberculosis was in fact only mild, but that the psychological stress to which he had been

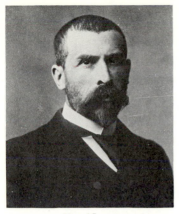
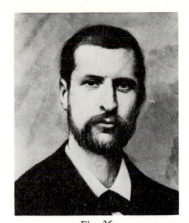

Fig. 35.   *Fig. 36.*

Fig. 35. Emile Roux (1853–1933).

Fig. 36. Alexandre Yersin (1863–1943).

submitted had been the cause of most of his symptoms. In some of his autobiographical notes about this unhappy incident, he wrote somewhat pathetically, yet very understandably, 'when I felt so miserable and forsaken during the time with Gerhardt, I often stood before the cupboard in which my collection of dyes was stored and said to myself, "These are my friends which will not desert me"'.

After two years abroad he recovered his health and returned to Berlin in 1889. He first set up in a private laboratory, but before long, Robert Koch, who by now had become Director of the Institute for Infectious Diseases, offered him a post there. Ehrlich was delighted and it was here that the next phase of his life began, during which he was to make a notable contribution to work which was being done at that time in the treatment of diphtheria.

The fact that a patient suffering from a contagious disease is feverish, weak, listless and without appetite suggested to early observers that, when bacteria attack a part of the body, they not only cause local damage but also liberate a poison which circulates throughout the body. Loeffler, who identified the diphtheria bacillus under the microscope, suspected that these organisms produced a poison in the blood, but it was Roux and Yersin, in 1886, who proved that such a toxic substance actually existed. They cultured diphtheria

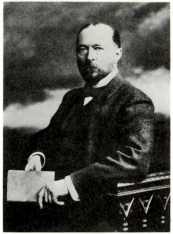
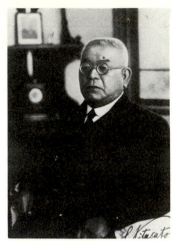

Fig. 37.   Fig. 38.

Fig. 37. *Emil von Behring (1854–1917).*
Fig. 38. *Shibasaburo Kitasato (1856–1931).*

bacilli in broth, then filtered off the bacteria from the broth. This broth, on injection into animals, proved fatal, showing that it contained a toxic substance. This discovery alerted people to the possibility that other organisms might produce a similar poison but only two other bacteria have been found to behave in this way, one being the tetanus bacillus. In 1890, von Behring and Kitasato demonstrated the presence of toxin in a broth culture of tetanus bacilli by showing that broth in which these bacilli had been grown, after filtration, produced tetanus in animals susceptible to this condition.

The next important step was the appreciation that the body, as part of its defence mechanism, produced antitoxins to neutralize these toxins. Von Behring and Kitasato demonstrated that when toxin from tetanus bacilli was injected into a rabbit a change took place in the serum, with the production of a substance which had the effect of neutralizing the toxins. They were then able to show that a mixture of toxin and serum, from an animal infected with the disease, was innocuous on injection into other animals, because the antitoxin contained in the serum neutralized the toxin. Following this, they demonstrated that serum which contained antitoxin was capable of

protecting an animal exposed to a lethal dose of toxin. In addition
to this work on tetanus, in the same year, von Behring reported
finding similar antitoxins in diphtheria. It was now obvious, therefore, that, if a large amount of the appropriate antitoxin could be
produced, so that it could be injected in high concentration, it would
be a valuable means of treating a patient who had an overwhelming
toxaemia from diphtheria. It was at this stage that Ehrlich contributed to the problem. Von Behring found that he was not able to
produce an antitoxin in high enough concentration to be effective.
Ehrlich showed that he could do this by repeated injections of toxin
into the blood of horses. He also devised a method by which the
amount of antitoxin present could be accurately measured, and
later, he established a central institute in Germany where all antitoxin used for treatment was standardized. For the first time therefore there was now an effective treatment for diphtheria. It was unfortunate for Ehrlich that his happiness about this achievement was
marred by von Behring, who tried to take unfair advantage over him
about certain financial arrangements associated with the production
of this antitoxin. This led to the irrevocable breaking of their friendship in a spirit of enmity and bad feeling.

The method was not so successful in the treatment of tetanus:
spores from tetanus bacilli lie about in the dirt and enter the body,
often when the skin surface has only been broken by minor cuts or
abrasions. This leads to an illness characterized by intensely painful
spasms of muscles, but the giving of antitoxin at this stage is useless
as the toxin will have already entered the body cells. It is valuable
however to give antitoxin immediately after any open injury, as a
prophylactic measure, because it will then be available to neutralize
toxin liberated into the blood stream, should infection with tetanus
have occurred.

Ehrlich continued to work at Robert Koch's Institute for Infectious
Diseases until 1896, when he was invited to take a government
appointment as Director of the State Institute for the Investigation
and Control of Sera, which was due to be opened in Steglitz, a suburb
of Berlin. The main purpose of this establishment was to enable
the Prussian government to establish a tight control over the production of anti-diphtheria serum and other newly found sera.

Ehrlich was delighted with his post, as he knew he would have a free hand with the work there and it meant that his long felt ambition to become head of a medical research unit, had at last been fulfilled. The buildings, however, were primitive, his laboratory was a dilapidated disused bakehouse, and the money available to him for research was limited and strictly controlled by a niggardly state budget. His enthusiasm and drive were immense and, in spite of these limitations, he and his assistants carried out important experiments on the effect of various chemicals injected into animals.

His work was so successful and he published such a large number of original papers in the medical journals, that Dr Altoff, the Director of the Prussian Ministry of Educational and Medical Affairs, felt that every opportunity should be given to this brilliant young investigator. Therefore, he approached the Lord Mayor of Frankfurt for help in improving Ehrlich's working conditions. Between them they succeeded in bringing about the foundation of the Institute for Experimental Therapy, which was opened in 1899, with Ehrlich as Director. It is obvious that such an institute would never have been built had it not been for the fact that Ehrlich had already shown remarkable progress in the application of chemistry to medical treatment. From the day of starting in this new institute, he had sixteen more years of life left to him, during which he made most of his greatest discoveries. It was a large and imposing building in south Frankfurt, near the hospital, with well equipped laboratories, library and reading rooms. It was an ideal environment for Ehrlich to develop the ideas on which he had already started working in Koch's laboratory and at Steglitz. The main principle of these ideas was based on his so-called 'side-chain' theory which was that, whenever there is infection with bacteria, various antibodies appear in the blood as part of the natural defence mechanism and, because of a specific affinity, become anchored by a side chain to the invading organisms, thus rendering them harmless. These antibodies behave in other words, like modern guided missiles and, indeed, Ehrlich often referred to them as magic bullets. He felt that, just as these substances are made inside the body for this purpose, it should be possible to make similar ones in the laboratory which, on being taken into the body, would poison the cells of bacteria, while having little effect on the normal cells of the body. He realized that such chemicals would be bound to have some toxic effect on the tissue cells and that it would be necessary to produce many different derivatives of substances, by altering their basic molecular structure, until one was found which would have a poisonous effect on bacteria with only a minimal effect on normal cells. He once tried to explain this theory, which was to guide him in his search for suitable anti-bacterial substances, to two English professors, Sir Almroth Wright and William Bullock, while they were travelling back from some conference, on the night train from Berlin to Frankfurt. He became so excited and carried away by his denouncement of his critics and by the elucidation of his theories, that the guard threatened more than once to turn all three of them off the train! Ehrlich had not only worked himself up into a state of feverish excitement, but had had a similar effect on his friends, who could see that it might well prove possible that this man, by his zeal and great knowledge of chemistry, could bring about a revolution in medical treatment. This in fact he did with the help of a team of workers, who with infinite patience, made hundreds of different chemicals and tried them out on countless animals artificially infected with many different types of disease.

He was a determined and somewhat autocratic director who insisted that his juniors carried out their allotted tasks as planned by him. He would not tolerate opposition or wilful evasion of his instructions by his staff, and if a man did not agree with his methods he had to resign. Although a hard taskmaster who expected those around him to achieve the same high standard as he set himself, he is said to have been at the same time friendly, jovial and very approachable. He was very fond of music and derived much pleasure from listening to all the popular tunes of the day played for him by a man who stopped his barrel organ outside his laboratory window. In addition he was always most helpful, kind and generous to those in trouble. It is known that he gave large sums of money to many people in distress or difficulty; he always found it difficult to refuse help and because of this people attempted to take advantage of such a kindly and sensitive soul. There were many times when he was left short of money himself because of the frequent demands of other people.

It was in this happy atmosphere that Ehrlich and his team zealously devoted their time to finding bacterial poisons. He was guided in this by experience gained from some of his other work. His study of anti-bodies and antitoxins produced inside the body, had led him to believe that similar chemicals might be found outside the body, which on ingestion would kill bacteria. His work with dyes and his observation that each one had a specific affinity for certain tissues, led him to the idea that it might be from similar substances that he could find chemicals which would be specially attracted to bacterial cells and would thus act as 'magic bullets', in a similar way to the chemical antibodies manufactured in the body.

The first chemicals with which he experimented in his search for antibacterial substances were therefore dyes. These were prepared, under the direction of Dr Ludwig Benda, at the Cassella Chemical Works in Frankfurt, which later became the famous I.G. Farben-industrie. Among the dyes first tested were Trypaflavine, and Trypan red. They were injected into animals which had been inoculated with a variety of different disease-producing organisms. It was found that they were particularly effective against the germs responsible for sleeping sickness. This is a serious and, without treatment, usually fatal disease which affects the natives of Africa. Trypan red, which was most potent experimentally, was therefore tried out in the tropics and found to be successful in the treatment of patients with this disease. It is of great interest that Ehrlich's particular approach to his search for chemotherapeutic substances led him to gain his first success with a disease which was a scourge to people thousands of miles from his own land.

His second success, and the great triumph of his life, was when he discovered a chemical which killed the organisms responsible for syphilis. Syphilis had been a world-wide problem for many centuries. It was well recognized that it was a disease contracted during sexual intercourse which started with a small ulcer, usually on the genitalia, and that the infection spread from there to affect many organs of the body, including the brain and heart, so that the patient could ultimately become blind, paralysed, mad, or die from heart failure. In view of the serious consequences of this disease many remedies had been devised throughout the ages but the only one which had been found to have any real effect was mercury rubbed into the skin. This proved however to be of limited value and to have side effects which at times were almost as bad as the disease. The widespread enthusiasm which greeted Ehrlich's triumph when he at last gave the world a drug which was effective as well as safe, needs little imagination. It was not however found by chance, but by tedious, dogged and persistent systematic trial of hundreds of chemical substances used on thousands of animals.

Ehrlich himself was fond of saying that in order to obtain success in research four big 'G's were needed: Geduld, Geschick, Geld, and Gluck (patience, ability, money and luck). He was helped in his animal work by two young workers from Japan sent to train under him by Professor Kitasato in Tokyo. Kitasato had studied in Europe himself and worked with Ehrlich when he was at the Robert Koch Institute in Paris. When he returned to Tokyo he founded an Institute which he modelled on the Pasteur Institute and called 'The Tokyo Institute for Infectious Disease'. It was from here that he sent certain of his most promising young pupils to receive further training in Europe.

The first one sent to Ehrlich was Dr Shiga, who arrived in Germany in 1902 and stayed until 1905. During this time the success with Trypan red was obtained and it was through this promising result that Ehrlich was able to interest a wealthy widow, Frau Speyer, in his work. Her generosity was such that she paid for the construction of a large new building adjacent to the Serum Institute, to be used exclusively for Ehrlich's chemotherapeutic research work. In addition she provided sufficient money to pay the current expenses of the work. Thus provided with the third of his four big 'G's (Geld) he was able to extend his work considerably.

Soon after work started in the Georg Speyer Haus, Ehrlich turned his attention to an examination of arsenic and its derivatives. Workers in many parts of the world were examining the therapeutic effects of this substance at the beginning of this century. Thomas and Breinl in Liverpool discovered, in 1906, that a substance called atoxyl, an arsenical compound, had a curative action in experimental animals affected with sleeping sickness. Unfortunately it was very toxic and liable to cause blindness by its effect on the optic nerve and

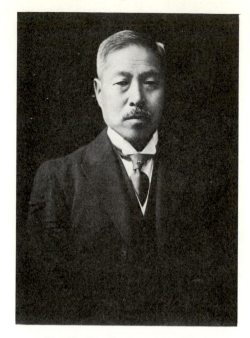

Fig. 39. Kiyoshi Shiga (1870–1957).

its use had to be abandoned. Most chemists concluded from a study of its chemical formula that it would not be possible to modify its structure, in order to produce a less toxic substance. Ehrlich decided to re-examine it, found that they were not correct and showed that it was possible to derive many other substances from it. With the help of chemists working under him, he produced altogether 606 different arsenical compounds, each of which was tested on experimentally infected animals. The one which showed great promise, once again against sleeping sickness, was No. 418—arseno-phenylglycine. Finally, Ehrlich reached his 606th preparation in 1907. His assistant who was responsible for the animal work at that time reported that it was of no use in sleeping sickness so it was therefore put on one side. Its true worth may never have been discovered had it not been that two years later, Professor Kitasato sent another young research worker to train under Ehrlich. This was Dr Hata, who for some years in Tokyo had been carrying out experiments with syphilis in rabbits.

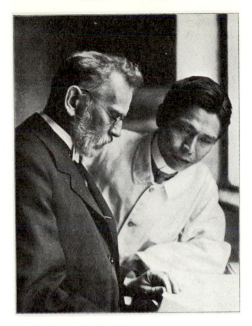

*Fig. 40. Paul Ehrlich (1854–1915) and
Sahachiro Hata (1873–1938).*

He started this work after the causative organism of the disease, which has the appearance of a spiral rod, hence its name spirochaete, had been discovered in 1905 by Schaudinn in Berlin. Hata now continued his work with Ehrlich and during the spring of 1909 systematically tried out all the compounds on rabbits infected with this disease. He was a tireless worker who patiently tested countless animals with numerous substances. He found No. 418 encouraging but continued and when at last No. 606 was reached, the results were excellent. As an adverse report about this substance had been given two years earlier, Ehrlich had it checked and rechecked before accepting his assistant's findings and allowing it to be used on human beings.

Ehrlich announced the discovery of this 606th arsenical substance at the Congress for Internal Medicine, at Wiesbaden, on 19 April 1910. He discussed the work which led to its discovery, Dr Hata described his animal experiments and Dr Schreiber of Magdeburg reported his clinical results in syphilitic patients treated with this new drug. The news was greeted by the Congress with great excitement and the Press, similarly enthusiastic, announced it to the general public in big headlines. The fact that the disease was widespread and crippling in its effect was reason enough for the public to have good cause to celebrate. What was possibly more important, was that Ehrlich had placed the search for antibacterial chemical substances on a scientific basis and had started the chain of discoveries which was to lead to the development of a succession of powerful chemo-therapeutic drugs in the twentieth century. He should not, therefore, be remembered only for his great discovery of a cure for syphilis, but also because much future success by other workers was due to the sound principles and methods initiated by him.

The world was quick to bestow appropriate honours on him. The Nobel prize had, interestingly enough, already been conferred on him in 1908, not for his work on drugs, but with Professor Metch-nikoff of the Pasteur Institute, for their work on immunity. After substance 606 was announced, universities throughout the world conferred honorary academic degrees upon him, the Prussian government made him a Privy Councillor with the title of Excellency, and the street in which his Institutes were situated, had its name changed from Sandhoff Strasse to Paul Ehrlich Strasse. All this naturally pleased him but what perhaps gave him the greatest joy was that he was elected to the very exclusive honorary membership of the German Chemical Society.

As soon as the Congress at Wiesbaden was finished visitors flocked to the Serum Institute to see Ehrlich. Patients afflicted with the disease travelled from all parts of the world asking to be cured. There were so many he could not possibly treat them himself, so he referred them to doctors who were interested in trying out the drug. These doctors were so numerous that he considered that it was fairest to give a small supply of the drug to each who asked, provided that in return he promised to report on the progress of his patients. Ehrlich also laid down strict instructions as to the method whereby the drug should be given, and stipulated that it was only to be used on cases in the early stages of the disease. As supplies at that time were strictly limited, perhaps it would have been better if he had reserved the drug for use in a few centres. By that method, carefully selected clinicians could have worked out the difficulties in the clinical use of the drug, established the best dosage and made a proper assessment of its curative power, by comparing it with a similar series of cases left untreated. This procedure is now common, for it is realized that it is the only way to assess quickly and efficiently the value of a new drug, but Ehrlich was having to deal with a problem which the medical profession had never before had to face. His method, although seemingly fair, led to a great deal of confusion and made it very difficult for him to supervise the effects of treatment. The drug could not be given by mouth but had to be injected into a muscle, which was unfortunate as most doctors at that time had little experience of the technique. Some doctors injected the substance into the superficial tissues under the skin, which caused pain, others dissolved the drug in water which had not been properly sterilized, so that infection with abscess formation developed at the site of the injection. These complications eventually led Ehrlich to insist that the drug should always be given into a vein. This was technically more difficult but he argued that it would be much safer, because any germs carelessly injected with the drug would be overcome by the defence mechanism in the blood stream. It was thought that, as this method would be more difficult for the doctors, they might not obey him, but it is of interest to note that it was generally adopted, clearly showing the high esteem in which he was held and the greatness of his authority.

The full chemical name of this 606th arsenical substance, or '606' as it was called, was dioxydiaminoarsenobenzol dihydrochloride. Obviously, it was neither possible to expect people to use this name every time they wished to refer to the drug, nor was it satisfactory for it only to be known as '606'. It therefore became known as arsphenamine, or by the trade name of Salvarsan.

A further medical congress was held the same year, this time at Königsberg, to enable all those who had been using Salvarsan to meet to discuss their results. During the five months since the congress at Wiesbaden, much work with the drug had been done and many very successful results had been obtained.

Ehrlich became involved in an incident, which on reflection is amusing, but which nearly prevented him from attending the conference. He loved Königsberg and decided, before going to the Conference Hall, to explore the city. He misjudged the time and arrived at the congress just after the doors had been closed. He tried many side doors but without success and therefore returned to the main door and knocked loudly. The scene which ensued is well reported by his secretary, Miss Marquardt, in her biography of the great man. She says that the knocking brought along a big, dignified doorkeeper, who opened the door sufficiently to look down upon the little man outside and said, 'What do you want...Sir...?', 'Everything here is full up', and he tried to close the door again. Ehrlich however pushed and cried out loudly, 'I must get in, I must, I must get in!' The doorkeeper became angry and started to push him away, 'It is absolutely impossible, I have told you already, the hall is quite full', he shouted. The noise, by this time, had attracted the attention of some of the doctors attending the Congress, who came out to see what was happening. By now, Ehrlich had pushed the door open wide enough to get part of his body inside. 'It is this obstinate little fellow who is determined to get in', the man said. Ehrlich of course was immediately recognized by the doctors, '...but that is a very great man' one cried out, 'that is Ehrlich himself!' One can well imagine the effect this had on the poor, unfortunate doorkeeper. Ehrlich was triumphantly welcomed and enthusiastically cheered by all those present.

Following Ehrlich's pioneer discoveries, many workers adopted his methods in an attempt to discover chemical substances capable of killing disease-producing bacteria inside the body. One man who was to have outstanding success in this field was Gerard Domagk, a German, who started medical research work after the First World War. His initial efforts were not particularly successful but eventually he showed such promise that in 1927, at the age of twenty-nine, he was appointed Director of Experimental Pathology and Bacteriology, at the Elberfeld Laboratories of the large firm of I.G. Farbenindustrie. This great commercial firm was able to give all possible financial help and necessary equipment to extend his search as widely as possible.

As by this time thousands of chemical substances had been pre-

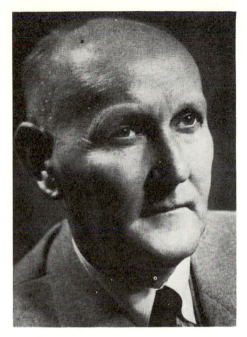

Fig. 41. Gerard Domagk (1895–1964).

pared in the laboratory, it might seem at first, that it must have been difficult for him to know where to start. However, he was strongly influenced by Ehrlich's success with aniline dyes and decided to explore further this group of chemical substances. Domagk was trained as a bacteriologist, so he sought the collaboration of two organic chemists, Mietzsch and Klarer, who at his request prepared a large number of azo dyes (dyes which have two linked nitrogen atoms in their molecule). He decided to study these because Eisenberg, in 1913, already had had limited success with one, a yellow dye called Chrysoidin. This killed bacteria in the laboratory, but its effect inside the body was disappointing. An even more important step had been taken in 1909, although at that time it seemed quite unrelated to the discovery of drugs, when Hörlein and others engaged in the production of new dyes for textile purposes, found that dyes were far more efficient if they contained a certain chemical combination—SO_2NH_2—the sulphonamide group. Such dyes were shown to be superior to any others because of their high degree of fastness to washing, which was produced by their extremely firm adherence to cell fibres. Mietzsch and Klarer, in the course of synthesizing hundreds of dyes therefore decided to prepare one which contained a sulphonamide group. Domagk tested this on mice infected with streptococci and found it to be extremely effective. Thus, it seemed that some property, which made the sulphonamide-containing dyes adhere firmly to textiles, caused them to behave similarly with bacteria and in so doing killed them. Therefore, he gave instructions that several substances containing this sulphonamide group should be made in order to find the one which was most effective. During the course of this search, his two chemists reviewed the various dyes already produced and decided to examine Chrysoidin which had shown such promise in 1913. In 1932 they attached a sulphonamide group to this dye to form a new chemical compound; when Domagk tested it on infected animals, the results far excelled those with any previous substance. The world knew nothing about this discovery for a further three years, until Domagk and his workers had submitted it to very carefully controlled trials. At first, it might appear that it was unfortunate that such a promising drug had to be withheld from sufferers with disease for so long, but it must be remembered that its exact therapeutic action, as well as any untoward toxic effects, had to be studied by carefully performed animal experiments before it could be used to its best advantage in man. Experience has shown that much tragedy, including death, or serious disability from unsuspected side effects, as well as shattering disillusionment from hopes unfulfilled, has been caused by drugs announced to the world too quickly. Also, it must be remembered that the drug produced by these German workers was of an entirely new type and it is to their eternal credit that, impatient as they must have been to tell the world of their success, they refrained from this until all necessary preliminary work had been completed. It was thus in 1935 that the drug was released for general medical use under the trade name of Prontosil rubrum. Immediately, from all parts of the world, reports were published of its great effect in controlling diseases such as pneumonia and particularly infection with streptococci such as occurs in puerperal fever. This disease had remained prevalent in women after childbirth even though by this time meticulous hand-washing was always practised by medical students and doctors. In Great Britain alone it still killed about a thousand women every year. It had always been a particularly tragic illness because such women were usually otherwise fit and because it occurred just at a time when they had the added joy and responsibility of new-born children; therefore, there was great excitement when Colebrook and Kenny, at Queen Charlotte's Maternity Hospital in London were able to show that, by using Prontosil in women with puerperal fever, the mortality rate could be reduced from about 20 per cent to the astonishingly low figure of 4·7 per cent.

The medical profession now had a reliable drug with which to kill streptococci which cause, in addition to puerperal fever, other diseases including the one-time dreaded hospital disease, erysipelas, and the very serious disease of the tissues called cellulitis. It also had for the first time a powerful weapon to use against pneumococci which often cause one particular type of pneumonia. But there was the disadvantage that this red dye also had a poisonous effect on the cells of the body. It therefore had the somewhat paradoxical effect of making the patient feel better by overcoming the infection while at the same time making him feel ill by its toxic effects on the tissue cells. A remarkable discovery was made in France in 1936, when Trèfouel, Madame Trèfouel, Nitti and Bovet, showed that the structure of this red dye underwent change inside the body, with the production of a colourless crystalline material, called *para-aminobenzenesulphonamide*, and that it was this substance which was responsible for the death of bacteria. It was then realized that this chemical had already been synthesized in the laboratory, during the course of routine experiments, as long ago as 1908, but of course nobody at that time had any reason to test its action against bacteria. Ehrlich, in his quest for chemotherapeutic substances, had started with dyes only to find that his most successful discovery was not a dye but an organic arsenical substance, Salvarsan. Domagk, by following his example, started his search in the same way and dis-covered the highly effective red dye Prontosil, only to find that its powerful effect was not due to its properties as a dye, but because in the body it was changed into the colourless substance which is now known to the medical world as sulphanilamide. Since the discovery of this drug, scientists all over the world have been carrying out a process of molecular juggling in order to obtain others, similar in structure but more effective. This has been a long tedious business, because it has entailed replacing part of the basic structure with various organic groups, by a process of trial and error. There are many places in the sulphanilamide molecule where substitution may be made, so that countless substances have had to be tested but, by this painstaking process, many useful sulphonamide drugs have now been obtained.

The scientific world wished to show its appreciation to Domagk by awarding him the Nobel prize. This however was not to be, as is shown in an interesting paragraph in the *Manchester Guardian* of 15 December 1939 which stated 'Five Nobel prizes have just been awarded and their bestowal raises some interesting points. They are divided amongst six scientists, three of whom are German. The German Government announced at the time of the award of the Nobel Peace Prize to Herr von Ossietsky that henceforth, Germans would not be allowed to accept Nobel prizes, and according to the German Legation at Copenhagen, this ruling still applies.'

One of these Germans was Gerard Domagk. Denied this high honour by his government, he received however a much more personal reward as, in the early experimental days of Prontosil, he was able to save the life of his own daughter. She had developed a spreading cellulitis in her arm, after having pierced a finger with a needle. Every known method of treatment had been tried, without success, and it soon became obvious that the girl had not much longer to live when, as a desperate measure, some of the new and scarcely tried drug was administered. The effect was remarkable and it was not long before she made a complete recovery. It must be rare for a research scientist to benefit from his work in such a happy manner.

The sulphonamides, whilst of inestimable value in their time and still having a place in the treatment of urinary tract infections, have in general gradually been replaced by other antibacterial substances.

Another group of chemicals which, because of their close structural relationship to the sulphonamides, came to be examined for antibacterial activity in the 1930's, were the sulphones. Buttle, with his colleagues in Britain, and Fourneau and his co-workers in France, independently described the marked effectiveness of 4,4′-diamino-diphenyl sulphone or dapsone in combating streptococcal infections in mice. And when in 1940 Rist and his colleagues in France, and a year later Feldman and others at the Mayo Clinic in America, observed that this drug and its derivative glucosulphone (promin) have a certain amount of activity in combating experimental tuber-culosis in animals, the possibility of using these drugs in human tuberculosis was considered. Although their usefulness in the treat-ment of this infection in man proved to be very limited, the fact that the morphological and staining properties of the leprosy bacillus are similar to those of the tubercle bacillus led Cowdry and Ruangsiri in 1941 to observe the effect of glucosulphone on rats infected with leprosy. This was followed by clinical trials in human leprosy, which were so successful that the sulphones have for many years played an important part in the treatment of this disease.

Other drugs, including the old Indian remedies Chaulmoogra and Hydnocarpus oils, have long been discarded, but two recently discovered ones are proving of especial importance. These are clofazimine, a phenazine dye discovered in 1969, and rifampicin, which when first used in leprosy in 1970 had already established for itself an important place in the treatment of tuberculosis.

Advances in biochemistry over the years have enabled scientists to extend the search, first started by Ehrlich and continued by Domagk, for chemical substances which when ingested are capable of killing cells harmful to the body whilst at the same time leaving healthy tissue cells relatively intact. This has resulted in the discovery of several important drugs, some capable of destroying bacterial cells and others of destroying cancer cells. It was research started by George Hitchings in 1942 in the Burroughs Wellcome Laboratories in New York, and undertaken mainly because of its possible relevance to the treatment of cancer, that eventually led Hitchings and Bushby to make an important advance in the field of antibacterial chemo-therapy. It was whilst examining the properties of a group of substances known as the 5-benzyl-2,4-diaminopyrimidines, that they found that the ability of these substances to interfere with certain enzymes associated with folic acid metabolism conferred on them important antibacterial and antiprotozoal activity. They further discovered that the action of the most promising one, trimethoprim, was due to it being a powerful inhibitor of the enzyme di-hydrofolate reductase present in bacteria, whilst having little or no effect on the corresponding enzyme in tissue cells. Knowing that the sulphonamides work in a similar manner, with the *para*-aminobenzoic acid they contain inhibiting an enzyme associated with folic acid metabolism in bacteria, they decided to investigate whether trimethoprim and a sulphonamide together might potentiate each other's action. This proved correct and their combination of trimethoprim with sulphamethoxazole, known as co-trimoxazole, was released for clinical use in 1969 and has found an important place in the treatment of typhoid fever and brucellosis as well as being widely used in the treatment of much more commonly occurring respiratory and urinary tract infections.

Other synthetic antimicrobial agents discovered in recent years, which are also of value in the treatment of urinary tract infections, are nalidixic acid and nitrofurantoin.

This brief review of chemotherapy, the science of combating bacteria with synthetic chemicals, will now be followed by an account of developments in antibiotic therapy, the science of combating bacteria with substances derived from other micro-organisms.

7

MICROBES FROM THE AIR

The next important advance was the discovery that products of certain moulds were highly effective in killing bacteria. The first one to be introduced was penicillin.

Most people now know that the discoverer of penicillin was Sir Alexander Fleming. He was born in 1881 on a farm in Scotland, the third child of a second marriage which his father entered into when he was already sixty years of age. Alexander came to London at the age of thirteen, where Tom, an elder stepbrother, had already settled as a general practitioner and they and two other brothers lived together in a house kept for them by one of their sisters. Alexander's first task in London was to continue his education at the Polytechnic in Regent Street and later found work in a shipping company in Leadenhall Street where he was paid 2½d. an hour, while his two brothers worked in a factory producing optical lenses.

In 1900, during the Boer War, Alexander and his two optician brothers joined the London Scottish regiment. After his demobilization Alexander was unsettled and indecisive about his future. Chance, fate, or the forces of predestination according to one's philosophy, then played a strong hand in influencing events which were to lead him to become a bacteriologist at St Mary's Hospital and, thirty years later, to discover penicillin. First, by propitious timing just as he came out of the army at the age of twenty, an old bachelor uncle happened to die and left him £250 which he was persuaded by his brother Tom to use to study medicine. His future was then directed by three factors. He was undoubtedly a brilliant student, but in addition he was outstanding at swimming and shooting. He lived equidistant to three of the teaching hospitals in London, but as he had played water polo against St Mary's, and for no better reason than this, he chose that school to study medicine. After he qualified as a doctor he was given a post in the bacteriology laboratory there because, in addition to being a gifted student, he was also a crack shot! It happened that there was already on the laboratory staff a young doctor called Freeman who was most anxious to get new blood into the St Mary's Rifle Club. Fleming was planning to train as a surgeon but as there was not going to be a vacancy at St Mary's for some time it meant he would have to leave the hospital. Freeman therefore did everything he could to persuade Fleming to take up bacteriology and talked the Chief of the Department into taking him on to the laboratory staff. The chief was Sir Almroth Wright, physically a big man, with a domineering, awe-inspiring manner, who held strong beliefs and was afraid of nobody, but was one of the most dynamic and progressive medical men of that time.

One of Wright's first posts had been at the Army School of Medicine at Netley Hospital where his main interest, as for the re-mainder of his life, revolved around the diagnosis and treatment of infectious diseases. Widal had shown that animals could be protected against typhoid fever by the injection of dead typhoid bacilli into their blood. Wright extended this to human beings and advised the War Office to have all men going overseas inoculated against the disease. The army authorities decided they would only allow it to be done on a voluntary basis and records were so inefficiently kept that it was impossible to carry out a proper follow-up of those vaccinated so as to measure its efficacy. Wright became completely frustrated and decided that it was impossible to carry out any useful scientific work in the army medical service, so resigned. Although this must have been a depressing time for him, it was to prove beneficial both to himself and to the world in general because in 1902 he was appointed professor of pathology at St Mary's Hospital. Here he had a much greater opportunity to do original work and to carry on his lifelong ambition of finding efficient ways of combating infection. He was appalled at the helplessness of physicians at that time to in-fluence the course of infectious diseases and stated publicly that the medical profession must find efficient means to combat infection as quickly as possible, or doctors would be forced to lose their status and become relegated to that of medical orderlies. This feeling was shared by many others and led scientists in various parts of the world to direct their energies to the problem. Metchnikoff, a Russian work-ing at the Pasteur Institute, observed that the white cells (phagocytes) in the blood engulf and digest bacteria, and Wright felt that the key to success was to find means to stimulate the action of these phagocytes. Scientists agreed that by artificial immunization it was possible to stimulate the natural defence mechanisms in the body, including the action of the white blood cells, as a protective measure against infection. Wright argued that the same process should be used to treat infection already established. This was much contested at the time but Wright was a born fighter and was determined to prove that this was the only way to overcome infectious disease. He expressed his views forcefully and at times aggressively but, in spite of this he was revered by those under him and was deeply respected by friends in many walks of life. Amongst them were the two famous scientists Ehrlich and Metchnikoff, and the dramatist, George Bernard Shaw. The latter often listened to Wright holding forth about his theories and based his famous play, *The Doctor's Dilemma* on them.

Fleming, in contrast to his chief, was a quiet, shy, retiring Scot, who would listen attentively to his master's pontifications, but say little. His rare contributions to a discussion however, although brief, were always penetrating and apt. He had a keen analytical mind and quietly sifted the evidence without being in a hurry to express his thoughts. He agreed with Wright that immunization was an important method of treatment but felt that this was not always sufficient. He knew that infection often overcame natural defence mechanisms in the body and that to rely on the stimulation of these processes was not enough. He had seen this demonstrated forcefully and dramatically in the 1914–18 war when he had written, 'surrounded by all those infected wounds, by men who were suffering and dying without our being able to do anything to help them, I was consumed by a desire to discover, after all this struggling and waiting, something which would kill these microbes, something like Salvarsan'.

It is obvious therefore that from an early stage Fleming was looking for drugs such as had been found by Paul Ehrlich; in this, he was to obtain no help or encouragement from his chief who was almost fanatically opposed to the idea of chemical poisons. Wright had said in 1912, when addressing the Medical Research Club, that 'to use chemotherapy against bacterial infections in human beings will never be possible'. His experiences during the war did nothing to alter

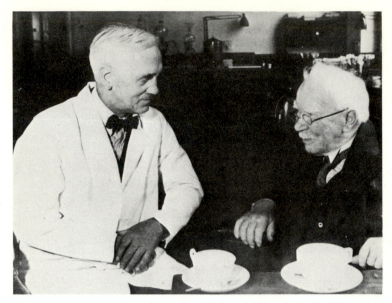

Fig. 42. Alexander Fleming (1881–1955) left and Almroth Wright (1861–1947).

this view; the antiseptics available at that time, which included carbolic acid, boric acid and hydrogen peroxide, could kill bacteria outside the body but were useless against infections in wounds. They did in fact more harm than good by damaging the tissues, while at the same time giving the surgeon such a false sense of security that he became less radical and less careful in his treatment of a wound. Wright spoke forcefully about this at the time and it obviously affected his judgement for the rest of his career. He influenced those working round him and Fleming, in a Hunterian lecture in 1919, remarked that during the war opinions differed about the treatment of wounds. Some considered it more natural to rely on the body's own defences and to do everything they could to improve these, while others relied on antiseptic chemicals to poison the bacteria. He showed clearly that Sir Almroth Wright and those working with him adopted the first method. Fleming was not satisfied that the stimulation of the body's defence mechanism was sufficient and, although he appreciated that the antiseptics in current use were valueless, he was determined to continue the search for more suitable bacterial poisons.

It seems as if Fleming had an uncanny preconception that he would discover something important from the examination of old culture plates contaminated by germs in the air, which he left lying about in the laboratory. Most scientific workers would agree that it is better to keep a working bench neat and to tidy up at the end of the day so that work can be started the next day in surroundings conducive to accurate, precise and systematic work. Dr Allison, who was Fleming's colleague in the same department at St Mary's Hospital, worked like this, but Fleming teased him about his tidiness and grumbled at him for throwing culture plates away as soon as he had finished with them. Fleming always seemed to keep his culture plates lying around in an apparent jumble for weeks, although it must be admitted he always knew where to find everything. He seemed loath to part with any culture, and always before doing so examined it very carefully to see if any interesting phenomenon had occurred. It was as though he was expecting to find something important and felt that it would only be a matter of time before he did.

In 1922 he had his first triumph. He had decided to investigate the defensive properties of nasal mucus and for this purpose placed some mucus from his nose amongst a culture of bacteria. About a fortnight later he was busy one evening cleaning some culture plates which had been lying around, when suddenly he stopped because he noticed that although some large, yellow colonies of bacteria were growing as expected, there was also an area where there was no growth. He knew that this blank space was round the site where he had placed his mucus and from this observation he deduced that there must be something in the mucus which had inhibited bacterial growth. When he grew the same bacteria in broth in a test tube, the broth developed a cloudy appearance, but within a few minutes of adding some nasal mucus to the opaque suspension it cleared. Next he observed the effect of adding tears to a similar broth culture and obtained the same result. It was astonishing. After this Allison and Fleming spent much time producing tears by the painful procedure of squeezing lemon juice into their eyes and then testing the effect of the tears on various bacterial cultures. Not content with their own tears they sought donors and encouraged the laboratory workers to co-operate by paying them threepence a time! This unusual procedure was the basis of a humorous drawing in the St Mary's Hospital *Gazette* which depicted children going to the laboratory to be beaten by one attendant, while having their tears collected by another! These experiments however were extremely valuable as they showed that tears, as well as other natural secretions of the body, readily dissolved and killed certain bacteria.

As it was agreed that the substance present in these secretions must be an enzyme which dissolved (lysed) microbes, Sir Almroth Wright, who had an extensive knowledge of Greek and enjoyed constructing new words, called it lysozyme.

Fleming carried out numerous observations with lysozyme. He found that it occurred in a wide variety of tissues, not only in the respiratory tract such as in the mucus secreted by glands in the lining epithelium of the nose, mouth and trachea, but also in the blood, especially in the white cells. He also looked around at nature in general and found it in flowers such as tulips, buttercups, nettles and peonies; he found it in vegetables, an especially large amount occurring in turnips, but the richest store of all was in egg-white. Egg-white was such an easily obtainable and rich store of this substance that Fleming used it for many of his further experiments. He discovered that lysozyme killed most readily the various types of bacteria which are not harmful to man and that it had little effect on microbes which cause disease. He concluded from this that the only reason certain bacteria are harmless is because they are kept under control by this substance. In further experiments he showed that with a very high concentration of lysozyme, disease-producing bacteria were also killed. Elated, he felt he must be on the verge of finding a method to combat these harmful organisms. The medical world of that day however were not prepared for such a discovery, so that, when he read a paper to the Medical Research Club about the remarkable properties of this substance, it was all too obvious that nobody was interested and at the end there were no questions and no discussion. Fleming was naturally hurt but he had the quality of dogged determination to persevere in spite of the indifference of others, so with the assistance of Allison he continued the work and between 1922 and 1927 published five outstanding papers. He showed that lysozyme found in egg-white was sufficiently concentrated to kill most bacteria in the laboratory. The next problem was to extract and purify the enzyme so that it could be used in the body. He was able to extend the work with lysozyme when Elliott Storer, who worked in his laboratory, developed in 1923 what he called a 'slide cell technique' for the purpose of studying the effect of poisons on bacteria under the microscope. The method consisted of placing two glass slides on top of each other separated by five thin strips of vaselined paper, giving four equal compartments. The compartments were filled with blood infected with bacteria, the open ends were sealed off and the apparatus placed in an incubator. The bacteria multiplied in colonies which were easy to count in the thin layer of blood between the two slides. Fleming next put various well-known antiseptics in the compartments to compare their effect both on the bacteria and on the cells in the blood. He found that every antiseptic known at that time killed the white cells far more readily than the bacteria so that it was obvious that none of them was suitable for injection into the blood stream. On the other hand, when lysozyme was placed in the compartments, it was the bacteria which were killed while the white cells were left intact. This observation led Fleming to inject an egg-white solution into a rabbit's vein which markedly increased the bactericidal power of the blood. He now believed that he possessed a useful weapon against bacteria, but realized that he would have to wait for the day when it could be purified before he could use it on human beings. This did not stop him from continuing to make valuable observations. In 1927, when he wrote his sixth paper on the subject, he described how he had found that, by adding lysozyme to a suspension of non-pathogenic bacteria in blood, most of the organisms were killed; the few that survived were removed and allowed to multiply in blood in an incubator. A higher concentration of lysozyme was then added which once again killed the majority of them. The process was repeated on several occasions with the few surviving bacteria and in this way a strain of bacteria was produced which was totally resistant to an extremely high concentration of lysozyme. Fleming had therefore now turned bacteria which were initially harmless to man into organisms which might be pathogenic. He inferred from this that lysozyme in the body had originally been an all-powerful weapon against every bacteria but that over the ages, some organisms had become resistant to it and it was these which now cause disease in man; he realized therefore that some other substance would have to be found to kill such organisms. In the meantime he tried to get a potent, purified extract of lysozyme prepared at St Mary's but he was not successful; neither Allison nor Fleming was a chemist and it is today amazing to recall that at that time St Mary's Hospital did not have a single chemist or bio-chemist on the staff to whom they could turn. In 1926 a young doctor called Ridley, who knew some chemistry, came to work in Wright's laboratory and Fleming hoped that he might be successful but they were to experience disappointment. The problem was not solved until 1937 when two chemists, Roberts and Abraham, successfully purified it in Dr Florey's laboratory at Oxford.

Fleming's experience with lysozyme however was far from wasted. Perhaps the most important aspect of the discovery was that it was a dress rehearsal in which Fleming, as the principal actor, was prepared and groomed for his role in the far more important drama which was still to be unfolded. As will be seen when his work on penicillin is discussed, the pattern of events was strikingly similar— the initial experience with the contaminated culture plate, his immediate recognition that he had made an important observation, the cool reception and indifference shown by his contemporaries, his dogged determination, his failure to find a chemist to isolate the substance, his patience and persistence against seemingly insurmountable setbacks and his final vindication when a potent antibacterial substance was purified by techniques developed in Howard Florey's laboratory at Oxford. The sequences in the two stories was so remarkably parallel that, in the midst of his work with penicillin, he must have felt at times as if he were reliving the past.

In 1928 Fleming was asked by the Medical Research Council to contribute to a book which was to be entitled *A System of Bacteriology* by writing an article on staphylococci. In preparation for this article he decided to examine a large number of culture plates on which these organisms were growing. It was necessary to take the lid off each culture plate and expose it to the air for some considerable length of time while he painstakingly examined the contents. Then, as was his lifetime habit, he left the culture plates lying on his bench

—it was as though he knew instinctively that if they became contaminated with micro-organisms, including moulds, from the outside air something important might occur; although he pretended it was a nuisance when this happened, he always re-examined them most carefully. One day, while talking to his colleague, Dr Merlin Pryce, he removed the lids from some old culture plates and found that as usual several of them were contaminated with moulds. He said 'as soon as you uncover a culture dish something tiresome is sure to happen—things fall out of the air'. He paused and after a moment added 'That's funny!' The reason for his exclamation was that, although the growth of bacteria on most of the plates was normal, some staphylococci on one plate around a particular type of mould had stopped growing so that instead of forming large, opaque, yellow masses the colonies of bacteria looked like drops of dew. Pryce, noticing Fleming's eager expression said 'That's how you discovered lysozyme'. Fleming immediately took a piece of the mould and put it into a tube of broth; at the same time he placed the dish on which the mould was growing on one side to treasure for the rest of his life.

It might be said that this event which was to lead to the discovery of penicillin had been made by chance as Fleming had not been specifically investigating the bactericidal properties of moulds but his special training had alerted his senses to the significance of the phenomenon which he observed.

He soon designed experiments to examine the properties of this mould. He grew it on an agar culture plate which he then inoculated with various types of bacteria spread out in lines radiating from the mould in the centre. He found that certain types of bacteria grew profusely at the periphery of the plate but stopped growing at the centre around the mould, whereas the growth of other types was not affected by it. He was fascinated to find that it was those types of organisms responsible for diseases in man whose growth had been most inhibited by this mould. This was a very exciting and wonderful observation and the exact opposite to the behaviour of lysozyme which he had shown killed bacteria harmless to man.

The identification of the mould at first eluded him. He consulted books on the subject and concluded that it was penicillium of the genus chrysogenum but two years later Thom, the American expert

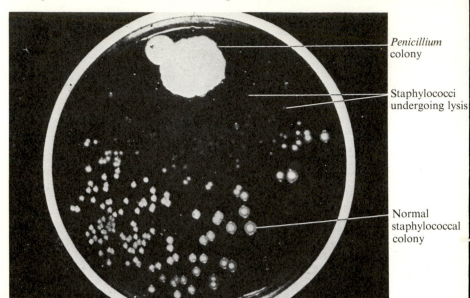

Fig. 43. Fleming's original culture plate (1928) showing a colony of
Penicillium *causing lysis of staphylococci.*

on moulds, identified it as *Penicillium notatum.* Thom pointed out
that this same mould had originally been described by a Swedish
chemist, Westling, who found it on some decayed hyssop. When
Fleming heard this he was immediately reminded of the remarkable
fact that David, in the seventh verse of Psalm 51 had prayed, 'Purge
me with hyssop and I shall be clean'—which he considered must
surely be the first known reference to its use as an antibiotic!

His next step was to culture the mould in broth, which at first was
not easy. Then he filtered off the mould and carried out tests to see
if the broth filtrate had any effect on bacteria. He did this by adding
the liquid to various cultures of bacteria and found that it contained
an active ingredient which markedly inhibited the growth of many
different types of bacteria. He decided to call the bactericidal substance in the broth 'penicillin' but, because he could not yet separate
it from the broth, he used the name for a time for the crude liquid.
He injected $\frac{1}{2}$ cc into a mouse and noted that there were no side

effects, and then injected 20 cc into the blood stream of a rabbit, finding it no more toxic than ordinary broth. He next irrigated large surface wounds in man and the human conjunctiva on repeated occasions without any unpleasant side effects. These experiments showed that this potent, antibacterial substance, unlike any substance previously used, did little or no damage to tissue cells.

His assistant with this work was a young man named Stuart Craddock, who was to become the first patient to receive penicillin. He suffered from an infected nasal sinus from which a profuse growth of staphylococci and some *Haemophilus influenzae* were grown. On 9 January 1929 Fleming washed out the sinus with this penicillin broth: the sinus was swabbed again three hours later and only one colony of staphylococci and a few of *Haemophilus influenzae* were grown which showed that even this highly diluted form of penicillin had been successful in killing off most of the bacteria. However, before it could be injected into the blood stream of man it had to be separated from the broth and purified. This was to prove difficult. First Fleming turned again to the young Dr Ridley who had attempted to purify lysozyme. As the broth could not be heated for fear of inactivating the penicillin, Ridley and Craddock allowed it to evaporate in a vacuum. This left them with a brown syrupy deposit which contained concentrated penicillin; but it proved to be very unstable, and its potency quickly diminished and vanished after a fortnight. Their aim had been to produce pure crystals of this substance, but they were badly in need of expert assistance and unfortunately none was available. This was a great pity because in later years when the problem was solved at Oxford, they realized how very near to success they had been. These two young doctors then parted when Craddock married and took a better paid job at the Wellcome Research Laboratories and Ridley, ill with recurrent boils, went on a cruise. On his return he trained to be an eye specialist.

Fleming however had faith and before long persuaded Harold Raistrick, professor of biochemistry at the London School of Tropical Medicine and Hygiene, to tackle the problem. He was assisted by a young chemist called Clutterbuck and a bacteriologist named Lovell. This team came up against technical difficulties and in the midst of the work Clutterbuck died; the others carried on but were baffled by the marked instability of penicillin. All their attempts to obtain it in a potent and purified form were of no avail and they were forced to give up the struggle. Naturally, Fleming was very upset for he had fully expected this expert team to solve his problem.

Lesser men would have accepted defeat, because, in addition to his frustration about the failure to purify penicillin, Fleming felt that his fellow doctors completely lacked faith in the substance. In February 1929 he read a paper on his observations with penicillin to the Medical Research Club, but his colleagues were as coldly disinterested as when he discussed the properties of lysozyme at a similar meeting some years previously. His own chief, Sir Almroth Wright, not only failed to encourage, but actively attempted to obstruct him. In June 1929 Fleming published in *The British Journal of Experimental Pathology* a report on the present position of penicillin, and stated as part of his summing up 'it is suggested that it may be an efficient antiseptic for application to or injection into the area affected with penicillin sensitive microbes'. He had to submit this article to Wright for approval before publication and his chief was not prepared to accept this conclusion. He pointed out that he had always taught that the way to conquer infection was to stimulate the natural defence mechanisms of the body, and that Fleming himself had shown that antiseptics did more harm than good. He ordered the paragraph to be deleted but Fleming, not deterred, was prepared to fight for his belief and, although a quarrel ensued, the paragraph remained.

Gerard Domagk's discovery in 1932 of the red dye Prontosil must have been a great encouragement to Fleming. It clearly showed that an antibacterial drug could be used safely and effectively in the body, but at the same time it must have made him unhappy to think that his own substance had proved so unstable and difficult to purify. To add to his frustration he found that, when he compared the effect of the new drug from Germany with penicillin on cultures of streptococci, penicillin was very much more active. He was therefore more than ever determined to obtain a pure form of penicillin. In the meantime, Prontosil and its sulphonamide derivatives made a remarkable contribution to medicine.

As Fleming saw the wonderful results of these drugs, he might have been tempted to give up the seemingly fruitless search for ways to purify penicillin, but he knew from observations both on patients and in his laboratory, that the sulphonamides were not effective against all bacteria and that, in some cases, bacteria initially sensitive to the drug had later become resistant. His hunt for a skilled chemist therefore continued and in 1934 a biochemist named Holt attempted the task of purification but without success. Meanwhile Fleming kept his enthusiasm going by talking to his friends about his discovery. One of these was Douglas MacLeod, the gynaecologist. In 1936, during lunch, the remarkable effect of Prontosil on puerperal fever was discussed—Fleming gave much credit to the new drug but told MacLeod that he had got a substance which was much better. The fact that MacLeod, working at his own hospital, had to admit that he knew nothing about this new substance, not even its name, showed clearly what little impact Fleming's discovery had made on his colleagues. He was not upset, but with his characteristic patience and enthusiasm, discussed its potentialities just as he did at clinical meetings. The difference though was that, whereas at meetings no one bothered to ask questions, MacLeod was impressed and spent much time talking to him. Occasions like this gave Fleming much encouragement, but when about this time he asked the professor of pharmacology at St Mary's to undertake the task of extracting penicillin, he was again rebuffed; the professor showed a complete lack of enthusiasm and would not even try.

Fleming was one of the first to use Ehrlich's Salvarsan against syphilis and had followed up his patients over the years to find to his delight that they had remained cured. He predicted to Dr McElligott that penicillin would have a powerful effect on the organisms which cause both syphilis and gonorrhoea. He was later proved to be correct, but in the meantime McElligott observed the beneficial effect of sulphonamides in cases of gonorrhoea, and used to tell Fleming and Wright about this over tea. It was no surprise to Fleming for he had tested this group of drugs against gonococci in the laboratory, but Wright was maddened to think that an antibacterial agent had proved so powerful. He was certain that a vaccine would be more effective and was somewhat mollified by some experiments of Fleming with infected mice which showed that a combination of a sulphonamide and vaccine was more effective than using a sulphonamide alone. This fortunately kept the relationship between the two of them happy but there is no doubt that Wright's antagonism towards antibacterial substances delayed progress. He took no interest in sulphonamides, treated the discovery as though it had never happened and at the same time closed his mind to the possibilities of penicillin. This did not deter Fleming and in 1936, at the second International Congress of Microbiology, he demonstrated the powerful effect of penicillin on laboratory cultures of bacteria, but nobody, sad to say, showed much interest. It is possible that his dry, reserved manner and somewhat diffident mode of speech contributed to this. Although his work was not recognized in his own country, it was receiving attention in America and when he attended the third International Congress of Microbiology in New York the famous bacteriologist, Dr Dubos, asked him what had become of that promising substance called penicillin. Fleming had to confess that repeated attempts to purify it had failed and that it looked as if it wasn't worth much. At the same Congress he met another American doctor, Alvin F. Coburn, who asked many questions about lysozyme. Fleming was delighted to find that people in America had taken notice of work which had received so little attention in England.

Meanwhile, work was going on unbeknown to him by Dr Howard Florey and his team at the Sir William Dunn School of Pathology at Oxford.

Howard Florey was born in Adelaide on 24 September 1898: his father, a prosperous boot and shoe manufacturer had emigrated to Australia from England in the 1880's, with a tuberculous wife and two daughters. After his wife's death he remarried and had two further daughters before Howard was born.

The boy had a very happy home life, and learning came easily to him so that by the age of twelve he had firmly resolved to devote his life to scientific research. In his 'teens he was forced to give up physics because of a lack of mathematical ability and spent his time exclusively on chemistry. Howard had planned to study this further at University and his decision to become a doctor stemmed entirely from the fact that his headmaster felt that the prospects for chemists in Australia at that time were limited. He had a brilliant undergraduate career at the Medical School in Adelaide, following which, in 1922, he sailed for England for postgraduate training in physiology at Oxford.

His ingenuity and originality in conducting animal experiments were quickly recognized by his tutor, the famous neuro-physiologist Sir Charles Sherrington. Sherrington was convinced that pathology, the study of diseases in the living, had for too long been based almost exclusively on examining the dead! – and for this reason in 1924 he encouraged Florey to transfer to the Department of Pathology at Cambridge, so that he might apply the skills he had acquired investigating normal animal function in the physiology laboratory in studying disorders of function in disease.

This approach to pathology as an applied physiologist rather than as a morbid anatomist remained with Florey for the rest of his academic life and led him to conduct numerous experiments on the dynamics of the circulation of the blood and lymph and to spend many years studying the secretion of mucus in the intestinal tract both in health and disease.

His first paper on this subject 'Mucus Secretion of the Colon' published jointly with A. N. Drury in 1928, surprising though it may seem, was the unlikely start to a lifetime's study of antibacterial substances. It was whilst he was contemplating whether mucus which lines the wall of the gut might form a protective barrier preventing bacteria which flourish in it from penetrating and infecting the wall itself, that he remembered that it was in mucus from the nose that Alexander Fleming, eight years previously, had found the antibacterial substance lysozyme. He therefore decided to study the distribution and antibacterial function of this enzyme in the mucus throughout the alimentary tract and published a paper on his findings, jointly with N. E. Goldsworthy in 1930. He realized however that any detailed study of its properties would have to be deferred until it could be purified. No one working with him at that time had sufficient technical knowledge, and indeed it was another six years before the task could be accomplished.

His postgraduate training, which lasted for ten years, included working in research departments not only at Oxford and Cambridge but also at the London Hospital and in America in Philadelphia,

Chicago and New York. In March 1932 Florey became Professor of Pathology at the University of Sheffield: the appointment of an applied physiologist to a Chair of Pathology occasioned not only surprise but a certain amount of criticism. Undeterred by this however, he quickly immersed himself in an ambitious programme of animal experiments designed to study various substances secreted into the gastro-intestinal tract. He was also anxious to have a chemist on his staff who could purify lysozyme for him, but he was thwarted in this by a lack of University funds. This caused him to feel very frustrated and he was delighted when in August 1934 he was appointed Professor of Pathology at Oxford, a post which he described as 'this magnificent job with all its opportunities'. His realization that any study of pathology must include an understanding of the complex chemical changes which constantly take place in all living tissues, led him to search around for some suitably trained young biochemist to join his staff. It was Sir Gowland Hopkins, the Director of the Sir William Dunn School of Biochemistry at Cambridge, who suggested that a young chemist, Ernst Chain, who had been working for his department since 1933 and had just completed his second Ph.D. thesis, would be very suitable. Chain, a Jew, born in Berlin in 1906 of a Russian father and German mother, had qualified as a biochemist but was forced to leave Germany to escape Nazi persecution on 30 January 1933, the day that Hitler came to power. On arriving in England he was befriended by J. B. S. Haldane who found the young migrant research worker a job in Cambridge. Chain never for one moment thought he would be staying in this country and was in fact planning to move on to Australia or Canada, so that his appointment to a permanent post with Florey at Oxford, led him, some years later, to say 'I was both extremely surprised and delighted, for I never expected such exceptionally good fortune to come my way in my unsettled condition, with a very uncertain future in front of me.'

Florey was quick to interest his workers at Oxford in the study of lysozyme, largely because he believed in its antibacterial powers, but also because he felt that in some way it might eventually prove to have a role in the pathogenesis of duodenal ulcers. He was delighted when, two years later, E. A. H. Roberts, working with him with the support of a Medical Research Council grant, obtained lysozyme in a pure form. Immediately this was done Florey suggested to Chain that he might like to study the antibacterial properties of this substance. This started Chain's interest in bactericidal substances in general and after completing his study of lysozyme, he went through the literature to see what other work had been done on this subject. He found a large number of papers dealing with antibacterial substances, and immediately became fascinated with the possibilities of microbial antagonism, or the destruction of one type of microorganism by another. He read a large number of papers on the subject, but the one which interested him most was that written by Fleming in 1929 on penicillin. He read that, according to Fleming, it could destroy dangerous bacteria and was free from side effects. Chain also read that attempts had been made to purify it but that these had so far failed. He was anxious to take up the challenge but first of all money was needed. The Medical Research Council in Great Britain was sometimes prepared to give small amounts up to about £100, but knowing that this would not be nearly enough, Florey and Chain decided to ask the Rockefeller Foundation for a few thousand dollars. Chain submitted a programme of subjects to be investigated and Florey was successful in obtaining an annual grant of $5000 for five years.

It was thus with American money that Florey and Chain started their investigation of penicillin in 1938. Chain had the task of isolating a purified extract from Fleming's crude mould, so that Florey could then study its biological properties. As Chain has pointed out since, the frequently expressed idea that the work was started as a contribution to the war effort is entirely fallacious. First it was started long before the war began and secondly, as Chain and Florey have both since admitted, they were in no way motivated by philanthropic ideals but entirely by scientific curiosity. As Chain said, in addressing the Royal College of Physicians in 1972,

That penicillin could have practical use in clinical medicine did not enter our minds when we started work on it. A substance of the degree of instability that penicillin seemed to possess according to the published facts does not hold out much promise for clinical application...The research on penicillin, which was started as a problem of purely scientific interest but had consequences of very great practical importance, is a good example of how difficult it is to demarcate sharp limits between pure and applied research.

It is clear therefore that Chain's ambition to obtain a pure extract from crude penicillin was no more than a scientific challenge to a biochemist faced with a natural product with unusual biological properties, whose instability up to that time had evaded the efforts of all those who had attempted the task.

Florey, with characteristic candour, also stated later in his life 'I don't think the idea of helping suffering humanity ever entered our minds.' Possibly, in saying this he did not strictly do himself justice because when his daughter Paquita suffered for some months from boils, he remarked to a colleague that there was need for a substance to combat the staphylococcus, the causative organism in this condition, and he must have been thinking of the possibility of using penicillin because he was well aware that Fleming had demonstrated that his mould could destroy this organism *in vitro*; also, whilst working at the Royal Infirmary in Sheffield, he had watched with interest C. G. Paine, a former pupil of Fleming, applying crude penicillin containing culture filtrates to wounds.

The first step was for Chain to obtain some of Fleming's original mould. This proved easier than he might have expected because by a curious coincidence there was already some at Oxford, which Fleming had sent to Florey's predecessor some years before for an entirely different research project. This had been kept and now came in useful, although Chain knew nothing about moulds and had to start from the beginning to learn how to handle them. His one advantage over Ridley and Raistrick was that the process of freeze-drying had been developed since their time and by subjecting the broth filtrate to this process he obtained a brown powder which contained penicillin with impurities. His problem now was to extract the penicillin from this. He tried to extract it with pure ethyl alcohol but failed, then to his surprise was successful with methyl alcohol and was able to obtain a small amount of partially purified penicillin. John Barnes, an assistant surgeon working with the famous Spanish surgeon, Trueta, at Oxford, injected it for him into the blood stream of a mouse without the development of any toxic effects. This was such an important finding that Florey repeated the experiment and was so surprised to find it had no effect on the mouse that he feared his injection had not gone into the blood stream. He therefore decided to repeat the experiment but to make this possible Chain had to produce more penicillin. This was no easy matter as his technique was still far from perfect, but it was well worth the effort as it confirmed that the partially purified penicillin was non-toxic. Further purification was obtained by Chain with the help of a young laboratory worker called Heatley and they set about testing its potency by placing it on culture plates adjacent to colonies of bacteria. These experiments showed that their partially purified product was one thousand times more active than crude penicillin. When eventually it was completely purified it was found to be a million times more potent than Fleming's first substance! They then devised experiments to test its effect on infections in animals. The first was on 20 May 1940 when three groups of mice were injected with three different organisms; half of them were given penicillin and half were not. Heatley sat up all night to watch with excitement as the treated mice survived while the controls all died. Next morning Florey and Chain were triumphant when they saw the result. They realized that they had in their hands an extremely valuable anti-bacterial agent which, if it could be prepared in sufficient amounts, could well make a major contribution to the recovery of sick and wounded troops. The war however was going badly, it was now June 1940, Dunkirk had fallen, and the possibility of imminent invasion of the British Isles confronted them. The Oxford team decided that they must save the miraculous mould and not allow the secret to get into the hands of the enemy: they therefore soaked the linings of their clothes in the brown liquid so that if only one escaped he would have enough mould on his person to start new cultures. In the meantime, they continued their experiments. On 1 July they injected a large number of streptococci into fifty white mice, half of them were given penicillin every three hours for forty-eight hours, the other half were left untreated as controls. Florey and his assistant were awakened by an alarm clock every two hours of the night. All

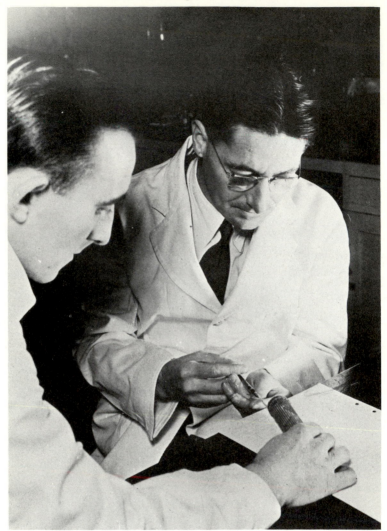

Fig. 44. Professor Florey injecting into a tail vein of a mouse.

twenty-five controls were dead in sixteen hours but twenty-four out of twenty-five of the mice treated with penicillin survived. It seemed almost a miracle but the result was reported soberly and factually in *The Lancet* on 24 August 1940. When Fleming read the report he was both delighted and surprised as he had no idea that this work

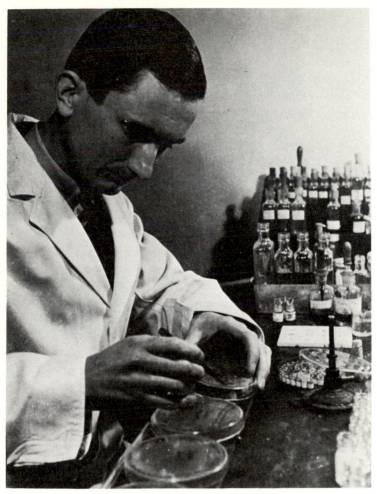

Fig. 45. Dr N. G. Heatley.

was going on in Oxford. He had asked so many chemists to purify penicillin for him, and their efforts had either failed or they had been too busy even to try. Now, when he had almost given up hope, it had been done for him without his asking. The Oxford scientists had been encouraged to do this work because of Fleming's precise accounts of the drug's potentialities in various published reports. They had not got in touch with him at any stage and, in fact, when

Fleming went down to Oxford to see him, Chain had the shock of his life because he had assumed he was dead!

It was obvious to all that the time had now come to inject the drug into the blood stream of a human being. The method of purification at that time however was such that only a small amount could be made and it was essential to increase production. This was a complex problem. Florey, realizing that they would now need outside commercial help, approached the directors of a well known and very large chemical firm. These industrial chemists considered the work carefully but turned it down as their factories were already fully engaged on war work already requested by the government. Thus they were faced with the fact that when they came to test the drug on a suitable patient only a small amount was available. In February 1941 an Oxford policeman was admitted to hospital seriously ill with his blood poisoned with staphylococci, an organism which had been shown in the laboratory to be sensitive to penicillin. A small abrasion at the corner of the man's mouth had become infected and from there the staphylococci had entered the blood stream to make him a desperately ill man with abscesses all over his body. The sulphonamides had proved ineffective and he was going downhill rapidly. On 12 February 1941 he became the first patient in the world to be given pencillin in the blood stream and, within twenty-four hours, improvement was so dramatic that a dying man had been transformed into a person whose illness was under good control. Although the organisms had been reduced in number they had not been completely destroyed in so short a time and the supply of penicillin was running low. A blood transfusion was given to help build up his general resistance, also a little more penicillin, but then the supplies ran out. The bacteria immediately multiplied and the patient's condition once again deteriorated and he died on 15 March. This was a tragedy because it was obvious to all concerned that with sufficient penicillin his life would have been saved. It was a failure as an experiment too, because, since a blood transfusion had been given, critics could say that any improvement was due to this.

After further supplies had been laboriously prepared three other cases were treated. Two of these were cured and the third died from a spontaneous rupture of a blood vessel after having been brought out

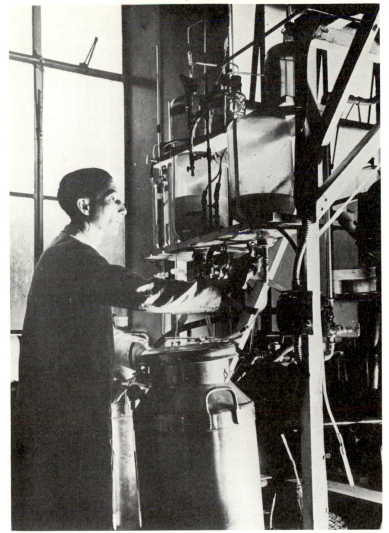

Fig. 46. Extraction of penicillin with make-shift apparatus at Oxford 1942.

of a comatose state by the drug. It was clear from these results that a remarkably powerful weapon was now available against bacterial infection but, before it could be put into general use, it was necessary to produce it on a commercial scale.

Florey approached many industrial chemists but none of the big manufacturers in England at that time were in a position to take on further work. Each one was at that time fully engaged on government contracts which had to be speedily completed because the country was in a perilous stage of the war. The only alternative was once again to ask help from America, but it was not sufficient now just to ask for a loan of money, it was essential to get American industry interested in wholesale production. This led Florey and Heatley, in June 1941, to journey to the United States with some strains of the penicillium mould. This must have been an extremely anxious journey because, they were not only exposed to the hazards of a sea passage in wartime, but also they had the worry of subjecting what was well known to be a highly sensitive mould to the intense heat of an American summer. In New York, Florey met Thom who eleven years previously had first identified the mould as *Penicillium notatum*. He was now head of the section which was studying moulds at the Northern Regional Research Laboratory at Peoria, Illinois. Thom introduced him to Dr Coghill who was chief of the Division of Fermentation and the problems which confronted the English workers were put before their American colleagues. It should be mentioned that at this stage all the British secrets which had been so patiently and painstakingly amassed were fully revealed so that the work could proceed as fast as possible. At no time did any of the British workers seek to protect their discovery by taking out a patent as everyone agreed that a substance of such vital use to mankind ought not to be the subject of personal profit.

The Americans decided that the first problem was to find a suitable medium on which to grow the mould. They happened to have a large accumulation of corn steep liquor which they had been using for other work and decided to try this as a culture medium for penicillium. It proved to be a lucky choice because they quickly improved the output by more than twenty times over the amount which had been obtained at Oxford and it was soon obvious that bulk production of penicillin would be possible. At the same time it was thought that there might be other types of mould which would give a greater yield. The army authorities were asked to collect specimens from all over the world but none of these proved to have any advantage over the original mould used by Fleming. In addition however the laboratory employed a young woman whose job it was to go to the local market to buy anything mouldy that she could find, so that she soon became known as 'Mouldy Mary'! One day she returned with a mouldy cantaloup melon and it was demonstrated that this mould, which was of the *Penicillium chrysogenum* type, gave a remarkably high yield of penicillin. It is of interest that it is from moulds derived from this original one found in the decayed melon from the Peoria market place that most of our penicillin is made today.

While Heatley worked in the laboratories, Florey travelled across America and Canada trying to interest industrial chemists in the large-scale production of penicillin. As America was not yet at war the task was easier than it had been in England and he managed to find two firms willing to produce large quantities of penicillin and to send it to Oxford for research purposes.

During the time that Florey was away in the United States, Chain continued to direct the work at Oxford and his team perfected a method of extraction which enabled them to build up a small supply of the drug. The first three casualties on whom it was used were some badly burned R.A.F. pilots at the time of the Battle of Britain. A small supply was also sent to Lieut.-Col. Pulvertaft, a bacteriologist in the Military Hospital at Cairo, for use on troops of the Eighth Army. The first man to have the benefit of it there was a young New Zealand officer suffering from widespread infection complicating a compound fracture of his leg. He had a high fever and was desperately ill with his sheets soaked with the pus which dripped from his wounds. When he had been ill for six months and was dying, small rubber tubes were put into the infected tissue in the left leg and a very weak solution of penicillin instilled. Within ten days the leg had healed and after a month he was back on his feet. Pulvertaft had enough penicillin for ten similar cases, nine of which made complete recoveries.

These were exciting and momentous days for doctors who had become used to watching men with badly infected wounds gradually succumb, in spite of all their efforts. Everyone was full of praise for this new substance and for the workers at Oxford who had produced it. It seemed for a time as if Alexander Fleming, whose sagacity and perseverance had made all this possible was to be overlooked and forgotten. His old chief, Sir Almroth Wright, however took the opportunity to compensate for his lack of enthusiasm in the early days, when he reminded the world of the man who made the discovery and to whom it owed an enormous debt of gratitude. This opportunity occurred after Fleming had saved the life of a friend who had been admitted to St Mary's Hospital seriously ill with an infection of the meninges—the membranes which cover the brain and spinal cord. This meningitis was due to an infection with a streptococcus which Fleming had demonstrated in the laboratory was not affected by sulphonamides, but was sensitive to penicillin. He therefore telephoned Florey to explain the situation, although the patient was comatose and the position seemed almost hopeless. Florey sent him a little of his precious reserve of the drug and on the evening of 6 August 1942, the first injection was given into the blood stream. Some improvement occurred but examination of the cerebrospinal fluid which circulates between the meninges showed that the penicillin was not getting to the infected part in a sufficiently high concentration. It was then decided to inject the penicillin for the first time through a needle directly into the man's cerebrospinal fluid. This was done with some trepidation as Florey had tried it out on a cat which had promptly died, but a similar injection into the man had no ill effects and he made a miraculous recovery.

This success caused great excitement, was widely discussed in medical circles and on 24 August 1942 *The Times* published a leading article entitled 'Penicillium'. It spoke of its virtue and pointed out that the substance was a hundred times more potent than sulphonamides but was difficult to make. It urged that in view of its importance every effort should be made to find methods of providing large quantities of the drug as soon as possible. It almost amounted to an order to the British government that, as part of the war effort, it should see that sufficient of it was made, but no reference was made to the pioneer work which was being done by the Oxford team, or to Fleming. Sir Almroth Wright may have lacked initial enthusiasm and been slow to give encouragement during the time that Fleming was studying the penicillium mould but, now that victory had been attained, he was not going to stand by and allow the world to reap the benefits of penicillin, without due recognition being given to the man who discovered it. He therefore wrote a letter to *The Times* published on 31 August, in which he pointed out that in the paper's recent leading article on penicillin it had refrained from putting a laurel wreath for the discovery round anybody's brow and made it clear that it was to Fleming that this honour was due. In view of the fact that he had been so hostile towards any suggestion that infection could be controlled by chemotherapy, it must have taken much moral courage to come forward, at the age of eighty-one, to support his junior colleague.

Fleming and Florey corresponded frequently and planned to mass produce penicillin in Britain. Fleming therefore went to see Sir Alexander Duncan, the Minister of Supply, who decided that a committee should be set up in Britain under the direction of Sir Cecil Weir, the Director-General of Equipment. On 28 September 1942 he summoned a conference at Portland House in London to include Fleming, Florey, Raistrick and representatives of chemical and pharmaceutical industries. Everyone attended in a most co-operative spirit and it was unanimously agreed by all concerned that the work must be done without any ulterior motive of personal gain and that all secrets must be shared so that the drug could be made available as quickly as possible for the treatment of the sick and wounded.

In the United States, progress was slow at the start, but all the workers were most enthusiastic and, before long, the technical difficulties had been overcome and large quantities were released. By 1943 sufficient stocks were available to supply the Armed Forces and by the following year there was plenty available for civilians as well.

Once large-scale production of penicillin had been started, it was not long before it was realized that four different types of penicillin were being produced. It was then discovered that one of these, known as penicillin G or benzyl penicillin, is the most active and that its almost exclusive formation can be ensured by adding phenylacetic acid to the culture medium. Commercial production has therefore since been restricted to this type and the names penicillin and benzyl penicillin have come to be used synonymously.

The pharmaceutical industry both in America and Britain realized that, in order to produce as much benzyl penicillin as was required, large numbers of giant-sized fermentation plants would have to be built. It was therefore decided to investigate the cheaper alternative of manufacturing the antibiotic synthetically, and for this reason a race began between different commercial companies and the workers at Oxford to see who would be the first to discover the chemical structure of the molecule. In 1943 Macphillamy, Wintersteiner and Alicino at E. R. Squibb, the American pharmaceutical company, took an important step forward when they crystallized benzyl penicillin and soon after a closely related substance was crystallized at Oxford. The task appeared to be so straightforward at this stage that Merck and Company were rash enough to wager a case of whisky that they would not only have the chemical formula but have synthetic penicillin within a few months. Events however were to prove this prediction very wrong.

Those working on the structure of penicillin at Oxford, including Sir Robert Robinson, Professor Wilson Baker, Ernst Chain, and E. P. Abraham, came to the conclusion in 1943 that penicillin must have a thiazolidine–beta–lactam ring structure. It was another two years before Dorothy Hodgkin, also at Oxford, was able to confirm the truth of this by the use of X-ray crystallographic analysis. The task took her a long time because of the relatively primitive calculators at her disposal, whereas today, with modern computers, she could have completed it in two to four weeks. The synthesis of penicillin, however, once its molecular structure had been determined, proved to be far from simple and in fact the chemical processes involved turned out to be so complex that it was not until 1957 that John Sheehan and K. R. Henery-Logan, working at the Massachusetts Institute of Technology and using what was for that time new and highly sophisticated methods, were able to produce synthetic penicillin for the first time. In spite of this painstaking and protracted work, the amount of antibiotic that could be manufactured by this technique was disappointingly small, so that the original biological production method of extracting the active principle from the mould of *Penicillium chrysogenum* has never been improved upon and remains the method of choice.

Benzyl penicillin remains to this day, in spite of the many anti-

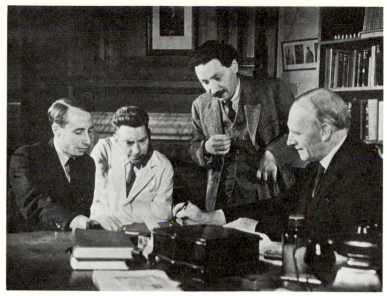

Fig. 47. Members of the group at Oxford who worked on the chemistry of penicillin. Right to left: Sir Robert Robinson, E. B. Chain, Wilson Baker and E. P. Abraham.

biotics since discovered, the best antibiotic against many strains of *Staphylococcus aureus* and in the treatment of *Streptococcus pyogenes* infections, pneumococcal pneumonia, meningococcal meningitis, syphilis, gonorrhoea, and the rarer gas gangrene, anthrax, and actinomycosis.

Fleming must have felt extremely frustrated at not being able to obtain penicillin in a suitable form for therapeutic use, because from his original paper in 1929 it is clear that he considered it would prove to be remarkably non-toxic when used in humans, having observed no ill effects from injecting a filtrate of his mould into both a rabbit and a mouse, and also from irrigating patients' infected wounds and the human conjunctiva with it. It is certainly fortunate that he never injected it into a guinea-pig, because it has subsequently been shown to have a uniquely lethal effect on this particular animal which if known initially would almost certainly have put a stop to any idea of it being used in man.

His belief in its freedom from side effects was not entirely warranted, for soon after it came into clinical use in the early 1940's, urticarial reactions simulating nettle rash were reported, and by the early 1950's there had been occasional incidents when the injection of the antibiotic had been followed by sudden severe shock, with at times fatal collapse. Time has shown, however, that life-threatening allergic reactions such as this are rare and that even skin rashes affect not more than 5 per cent of the population. It is in fact true to say that in comparison with most other antibiotics, penicillin is remarkably free from toxicity and it is nothing short of a miracle that it should have been the first one to have been discovered.

The world naturally hastened to pay homage to those responsible for the discovery of such a miraculous antibiotic. In 1944 both Fleming and Florey were knighted and one year later they shared with Ernst Chain the Nobel Prize for Physiology and Medicine. Professor Sir Alexander Fleming lived another ten years during which time he was able to watch the revolution in medicine brought about by his discovery. Florey and Chain were, of course, still relatively young men. Florey continued to serve the world of science with such distinction, his influence extending from experimental physiology to clinical medicine, to education, and to the country's scientific policies in general, that in 1965 he was created a Life Peer and became Baron Florey of Adelaide and Marston and the same year was appointed a member of the Order of Merit. He died in 1968.

Ernst Chain continued his work at Oxford as a lecturer in chemical pathology until 1948 when, frustrated at not being able to obtain what he considered to be adequate equipment and finance to continue his research on antibiotics, he left Oxford and became Director of the International Research Centre for Chemical Micro-biology at the Instituto Superiore di Sanita in Rome. In 1961 he returned to this county on his appointment as Professor of Bio-chemistry at the Imperial College of Science at the University of London, a post he held until his retirement in 1973; his outstanding contributions to medical science having led to a knighthood being conferred on him fourteen years previously.

This completes the story of how three men, from widely differing backgrounds, in their several ways and with the assistance of many colleagues both in Britain and America, made a contribution of such

importance in the fight against bacterial disease as to earn for themselves an immortal place in the history of medicine and the lasting
gratitude of all mankind. Their discovery was of outstanding value
not only because of the powerful action of the antibiotic itself, but
because, as prophesied by Florey at a meeting at the Royal Society
of Medicine in 1944, when he said 'some chemist will manipulate the
penicillin molecule to improve its performance', it has in fact since
proved possible to obtain from the parent substance a wide range of
other antibiotic substances each with its own special place in the
treatment of bacterial infections.

Some of the first to modify the structure of benzyl penicillin by
chemical manipulation were Behrens and his colleagues at the
research laboratories of Eli Lilly at Indianapolis in the mid 1940's.
Benzyl penicillin, as has been said, is produced by the addition of
phenylacetic acid to the medium in which the penicillium mould is
cultured. These workers added various other derivatives of acetic
acid and in 1948, by substituting phenoxyacetic acid, produced
phenoxymethyl penicillin or penicillin V. Its great advantage over
benzyl penicillin is that whereas the latter, being destroyed by acid
in the stomach, has to be given by injection, this substance, being
acid-resistant, can be taken by mouth. It is somewhat curious that
this important property was initially overlooked and not recognized
until 1953, when attention was drawn to it by Brunner, Brandl and
Margreiter in Austria. Since then it has remained the antibiotic of
choice in the treatment of *Streptococcus pyogenes* throat infections.
It is in fact the routine use of benzyl penicillin and, since its discovery,
of phenoxymethyl penicillin in this type of infection which has led to
such a dramatic decrease in recent years in the incidence of acute
nephritis and acute rheumatic fever, as both are the result of an
abnormal immunological response to this particular type of
streptococcus.

The dramatic effect of penicillin on serious, potentially lethal
staphylococcal infections quickly became apparent when Dr Charles
Fletcher in 1941 first administered the antibiotic to patients at the
Radcliffe Infirmary in Oxford, and this in spite of the fact that the
material used at that time was 99 per cent impure! This happy state
of affairs, however, was not to last, for by the late 1940's and early

1950's staphylococcal infections were spreading through hospital wards quite uncontrolled by the highly purified benzyl penicillin which by that time was available. This was not altogether surprising, for Fleming had recognized the occasional strain of *Staphylococcus* resistant to penicillin as early as 1943 and a year later the American bacteriologist Kirby showed that such strains are not only immune to the action of penicillin, but by secreting an enzyme actively destroy it. This was not however the first time that enzymic destruction of an antibiotic by bacteria had been recognized. Abraham and Chain had drawn attention to this phenomenon in 1940 when, observing that penicillin has little effect against Gram-negative bacilli, they wondered whether this might be due to such organisms secreting some biochemical substance capable of destroying it. They were able to confirm this hypothesis by crushing the cells of a strain of *Escherichia coli* and finding inside an enzyme which they called penicillinase. Subsequent work has shown that the penicillinase inside Gram-negative enterobacteria, and the one secreted by staphylococci, both operate by opening the beta-lactam ring of the penicillin molecule. It is for this reason that they are also referred to as beta-lactamases. These enzymes will be discussed more fully in the last chapter, but suffice it to say at this stage that by the mid 1940's their existence had been recognized and led Chain to contemplate whether by modifying the structure of the penicillin moleule, it might be possible to produce an antibiotic unaffected by staphylococcal penicillinase. The need for such a substance had certainly become evident by 1948, when Mary Barber presented data showing that in the hospital environment generally most penicillin-sensitive staphylococci had been eradicated, but that increasingly their place was being taken by penicillinase-secreting resistant ones, so that by that year over 50 per cent of the staphylococci in hospitals were penicillin-resistant.

Chain felt that in order to achieve any success in modifying the penicillin molecule he required large-scale fermentation equipment such as many commercial companies possessed, rather than the relatively small type of apparatus available to him at Oxford. It was because no amount of pleading on his part with the University authorities there would persuade them to provide him with what he considered to be adequate equipment that led him, whilst on a lecture tour in 1948, to accept Professor Domenico Marrota's invitation to become Director of the International Research Centre for Chemical Microbiology in Rome. The main attractions of the post were the provision of a sizeable fermentation plant, the installation of which was started in 1949 and finished in 1951, and sufficient funds for his research needs. Chain was aware that benzyl penicillin, the most widely used natural penicillin in medical practice, possessed a side chain phenylacetic acid, but that also other penicillins with different side chains occur in nature, and further that Behrens and his colleagues had shown that various penicillins could be produced by altering the type of acetic acid added to the culture medium used in the fermentation of *Penicillium chrysogenum*. It was their success in producing phenoxymethyl penicillin by the addition of phenoxyacetic acid that eventually prompted him during his time in Rome to produce *para*-aminobenzyl penicillin biosynthetically by adding *para*-aminoacetic acid to the culture medium.

In 1954 the directors of the British pharmaceutical company, Beecham, were encouraged by their Chairman, H. G. Lazell, to explore the possibilities of starting research in the field of antibiotics and turned to Chain for advice as to the best way to go about this. Chain informed them that it was essential for them first of all to build a fermentation plant costing at least £50,000, and whilst this was being constructed the firm, towards the end of 1955, sent two of its scientists, G. N. Rolinson and F. R. Batchelor, to Rome to work with him; it was during their stay there that *para*-aminobenzyl penicillin was produced.

On returning to England a year later, Rolinson and Batchelor quickly put their experience gained in Rome to good use when with, F. P. Doyle and J. H. C. Nayler, they examined the structure of the substance which forms during the course of fermenting *Penicillium chrysogenum* before any precursor acid is added. The Beecham team found that this substance, whilst chemically similar to penicillin, has none of its biological activity, but that as the addition of phenylacetic acid to it results in the production of benzyl penicillin, they concluded that it must be the nucleus or chemical core of the penicillin molecule. The existence of such a nucleus had, in fact, first been

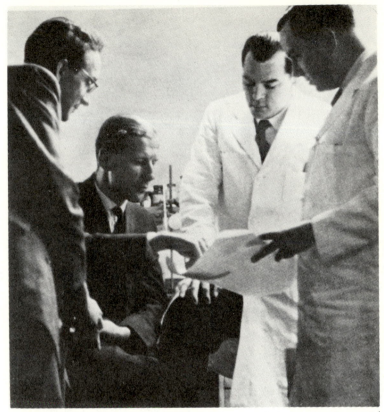

Fig. 48. Members of the Beecham team who identified the penicillin nucleus (6-APA). Left to right: Mr F. P. Doyle, Dr G. N. Rolinson, Dr F. R. Batchelor and Dr J. H. C. Nayler.

recognized in Japan by Sakaguchi and Murao in 1950 and by Kato in 1953, but the English scientists took the matter further by successfully analysing its chemical structure and announcing in 1959 that it is 6-aminopenicillanic acid (6-APA). This was a very exciting discovery and one of fundamental importance, as it now meant that chemists could at last manufacture many modifications of penicillin, each with its own characteristic properties, simply by the addition of various side chains to this nucleus.

Batchelor, Chain and Rolinson had concluded by 1961 that the extraction of 6-APA when produced by direct fermentation was

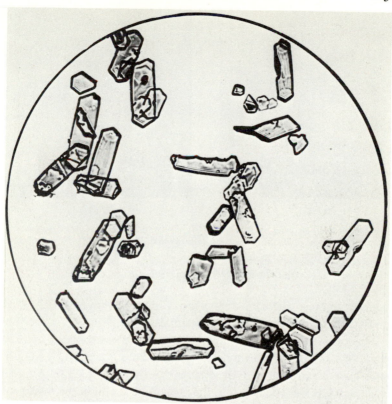

Fig. 49. A photomicrograph of the first pure crystals which were obtained of the penicillin nucleus (6-APA).

difficult and it was therefore a great step forward when these workers, together with M. Richards, announced that year that an enzyme found in various streptomycetes was capable of removing the side chain from phenoxymethyl penicillin with the liberation of 6-APA. Later, workers from the Bayer Research Laboratories and others, discovered enzymes capable of liberating 6-APA in large quantities from benzyl penicillin. This ready availability of 6-APA meant that by adding various side chains to the nucleus several thousands of semi-synthetic penicillins could be produced in the research laboratories of pharmaceutical companies all over the world. It is therefore much to the credit of the Beecham group that the small

The Battle against Bacteria

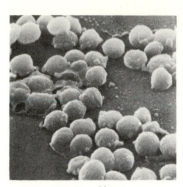
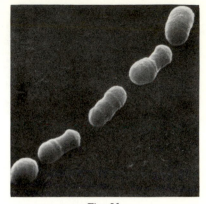

Fig. 50.   *Fig. 51.*

Fig. 50. An electron micrograph of Staphylococcus aureus *after exposure to ampicillin (compare with normal, Fig. 18, p. 35).*

Fig. 51. An electron micrograph of Streptococcus pyogenes *after exposure to ampicillin (compare with normal, Fig. 19, p. 35).*

number of these which have come into clinical use have all been made in that particular company's laboratories.

Two of these, phenethicillin and propicillin, introduced in 1959 and 1961 respectively, being acid-resistant may be taken by mouth, and have a range of activity predominantly against Gram-positive organisms. It was thought that they would be useful in the treatment of streptococcal throat infections, but in practice they are no better than the original phenoxymethyl penicillin (penicillin V) for this purpose.

The first major advance occurred in 1960 with the introduction of methicillin, an antibiotic which given by injection has the remarkable property of being resistant to the action of the penicillinase produced by staphylococci. About a year later it was replaced by cloxacillin which could be given by injection or by mouth, and in 1970 this in turn was superseded by flucloxacillin, as this is even better absorbed when taken orally.

The other outstanding semi-synthetic antibiotic produced by Beecham, and now probably the one most frequently used of all the penicillins, is ampicillin. The company, proud that it was a British discovery, marketed it in 1961 under the name of Penbritin. It is

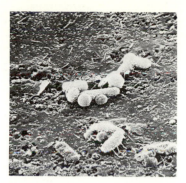

Fig. 52. An electron micrograph showing markedly deformed Escherichia coli *after only twenty minutes' exposure to amoxicillin* (*compare with normal, p. 37*).

somewhat less active than benzyl penicillin against Gram-positive organisms, and like this antibiotic is destroyed by penicillinase, but the fact that it is many times more powerful than benzyl penicillin against various Gram-negative organisms means that it has a very wide range of antibiotic activity and an important place in the treatment of commonly occurring chest, urinary tract and biliary tract infections. At the present time it is gradually being superseded by amoxicillin, another antibiotic produced by Beecham, with a similar structure but which is even better absorbed when taken by mouth.

One other semi-synthetic penicillin, carbenicillin, numbered 2064 in the Beecham Research Laboratories series and introduced in 1967, has the distinction of being the only penicillin with activity against the *Pseudomonas* and it is also active against all species of *Proteus* and certain other enterobacteria.

There are therefore at the present time a number of different penicillins, including benzyl penicillin and phenoxymethyl penicillin, both of which are produced biologically, and fluocloxacillin, ampicillin and carbenicillin which are produced semi-synthetically, each with specific indications and as a group having such wide-ranging activity that together they constitute a powerful force with which a very large number of highly dangerous disease-producing bacteria may be attacked.

8

MICROBES FROM THE SOIL

While young Fleming was playing in the fields around his father's farm in Scotland, another boy, who was to make a similar and equally important contribution to medical science, was growing up in a humble home in the isolation of the Russian Ukraine. His name was Selman Waksman. His birth on 8 July 1888 could hardly have been less propitious. His birthplace was the bleak, small town of Novaia-Priluka where the inhabitants lived in primitive, white-washed, straw-thatched houses. They were for the most part poor because, although the soil was very fertile and the crops plentiful, all the profits went to the landlords, the Czar and the police. It was a land filled with dissatisfaction, distrust and corruption. The peasants in Russia at that time had been liberated from slavery about forty years previously, but they still had much cause for bitterness, and the revolution was in the making. Waksman's family was Jewish and the Jews existed in a state of uneasy truce with the rest of the population.

Waksman's father had inherited some land but was not particularly industrious and although Selman liked him, they had no interests in common. His mother, on the other hand, was a bright, dynamic person who was his inspiration, and during his childhood they were devoted to each other. Their attachment was made closer by the fact that he was an only child, except for a brief period at the age of seven when he had a sister, who lived for less than two years.

He attended the local school and in addition his mother arranged for him to have some private tuition at home. He was quick to learn and by the age of thirteen, encouraged by his mother, he began to teach others and organized a school to teach children who otherwise would have remained without any education. For a time he lived a happy life at home with his mother, but this was not to last, because as he reached maturity the country was plunged into the disastrous Russo-Japanese war of 1904 to 1905. This had far-reaching consequences and awakened the people to a realization of their miserable

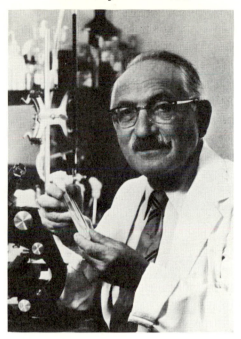

Fig. 53. Selman A. Waksman (1888–1973).

existence, and revealed to them how corrupt and rotten was their government and the extent to which they were exploited by the rulers. Organized protests and general strikes developed and the Czar was forced to promise improvements. No sooner had he done this than the police and cossacks raided the towns and arrested leaders of the revolution, shooting some and deporting others to Siberia. The suppression was ruthless and many innocent people lost their lives.

The little town of Priluka was not directly involved, but Waksman realized that the spirit of disunity which had split the country was bound to affect him sooner or later. He was therefore determined to complete his education as quickly as possible before everything became too disorganized. He left home to continue his studies in the bigger cities. Examinations were difficult because of the strong bias against Jews but his work was of such outstanding merit that the authorities were forced to pass him.

This antagonism to the Jews was expressed not only in everyday life, but also in the official attitude of school authorities. Many schools would only take a son of Jewish parents on condition that they not only paid for their child, but also for a non-Jewish boy as well. Jewish teachers too did not escape from this tyranny and one of Waksman's most successful teachers, a hunchback who taught mathematics, physics and chemistry, had to organize his own evening school because no university or school would employ him. This meant that he was deprived of laboratory facilities and could not give practical demonstrations in chemistry and physics, but he was devoted to his work and managed to hold the attention of his class with the help of a blackboard alone.

Waksman was nearing the end of his school studies when, without warning, he suffered a most grievous blow which was radically to affect his future. In the summer of 1909 while he was at home on holiday, his mother suddenly developed an obstruction of the bowel for which an immediate operation was necessary. This was only possible in a large hospital and they had to undertake an overnight train journey to Kiev. By the time she reached hospital, his mother's condition was too poor for her to stand up to an operation. Her son never left her, while for two weeks her condition gradually deteriorated. At her death he felt himself completely alone, for although his father and cousins were there, they were of little account.

He decided that he must move as quickly as possible from the neighbourhood where he had so many memories of his mother and, in the autumn of 1909, he and a friend returned to Odessa to continue their studies. In the following year he passed his final examination which permitted him to enter university. He was anxious not to go to a university in Russia, as entrance to these institutions for Jews was strictly limited, the country was becoming increasingly unhappy and divided, with the people living in fear of the Czar and his brutal police, while the future for Jews was particularly black. Above all, the one person to whom he was deeply attached had died, so he decided to emigrate and start a new life elsewhere. Some of his cousins had already settled in America and wrote persuading him to join them. He left Europe in the middle of October 1910 on his journey to the New World. He was over twelve days in the steerage accommodation of a small ship, where he shared a meagre diet of herrings and boiled potatoes, or boiled beef and black bread with several hundred other youthful emigrants. His boat arrived on 2 November 1910 in Philadelphia, where he was met by two of his cousins. One of them, Mendel Kornblatt, took him to his farm at Metuchen in New Jersey, where he stayed for some time. This cousin was to have a great influence on Selman's future. He showed him the problems of farm life, and gave him instructions in the basic principles of plant and animal growth, and the influence exerted on this by environment, nutrition and heredity. He taught him how best to prepare and use compost, the proper selection of seeds, the art of growing vegetables and the technique of rearing chickens. Waksman had a scientific type of mind and was delighted to find that his cousin was able to introduce him to all the fundamental chemical and biological aspects of agriculture. It encouraged him to want to learn more about the chemical reactions which occur in living bodies so he decided he ought to become a student at a university. At first he thought that he could best be trained in the subject at a medical school but at the suggestion of his cousin he visited Rutgers College, New Brunswick, only a few miles away from the farm. There he discussed his future with another immigrant from Russia, Dr Jacob Lipman, head of the Department of Bacteriology, and soon to become Dean of the College of Agriculture. Lipman persuaded him to apply for training at his college.

With the help of a scholarship gained in a State competitive examination he began work as an agricultural student at Rutgers in September 1911. It was not easy for him to work and compete with other students in this new country, with its language which was strange to him and its very different social pattern. He found the American students were not very helpful and at times laughed at his difficulties with their language, but he was determined to let nothing deter him. He was fortunate in having some inspiring teachers to instruct him in chemistry, physics, biology, bacteriology and all the various branches of scientific agriculture. For the first two and a half years at the university he continued to live on his cousin's farm. This had the advantage that he was able to earn his keep by helping with the work there but it did also mean that he was not able to read his books as much as he would have liked. He therefore moved to New Brunswick so that he could be nearer to the university, and to keep himself alive took on various spare-time jobs including teaching English to foreign immigrants. As his course in agriculture proceeded he developed a particular interest in the study of the soil and, as he had made extremely rapid progress during his course, he was excused from attending formal classes during his last year and was able to devote himself to a research project. The subject he chose was an enumeration of the different types of micro-organisms to be found in the soil. It was this study, initiated during his last year of student life, which was to lead him years later to the discovery of streptomycin. Nobody could have anticipated that such an important contribution to medicine would come from a study of the soil, and certainly Waksman's early interest was entirely academic.

In this study he dug trenches in the college farm each month of the year and observed that there were various quite distinct soil layers at different depths. He took samples of soil from each layer under aseptic conditions and cultured them on special culture media. He found that the most plentiful organisms were colonies of bacteria but that colonies of moulds or fungi were also scattered about. In addition, to his great surprise, he noted an abundance of small colonies which to the naked eye looked like bacteria but under the miscroscope had certain of the characteristics of moulds. When he drew the attention of his teachers to these he found that they did not know much about them. After further study Waksman came to the conclusion that they were representatives of what was then an obscure group of higher bacteria known as actinomycetes. It had been recognized for some thirty years that a member of this group is the cause of actinomycosis, a disease affecting both cattle and man and which is now treatable with the mould derivative penicillin. This is therefore a good example of the way man has learned to counteract the effects of one microbe by the action of a substance contained in another.

It was from various actinomycetes and the closely related streptomycetes that Waksman, and others at a later date, were to produce a wide range of important antibiotics. He little knew when his interest was first focused on them what an important part they were to play in his life, but for some compelling reason he found that he was to make a close study of them over many years, and that it was to remain his major scientific interest for the rest of his life.

He graduated with a Bachelor of Science degree in 1915. His teacher of botany, Dr Halsted, appreciated his abilities and offered him a post in his department. Waksman felt that his primary interest was not in general botany but in a specialist study of the soil and its life, especially in the little understood actinomycetes. This fundamental desire to study the mysteries of the soil must have been subconsciously developing in his mind since the days of his childhood spent amongst the highly productive fertile black earth of the Russian Ukraine, for every step he had taken since seems to have been directed towards this. So he turned down Halsted's offer and discussed his ambitions with Dr Lipman who had taught him soil bacteriology. As soon as Dr Lipman knew of his particular interest he was appointed as research assistant in soil bacteriology at the New Jersey Agricultural Experimental Station, an Institution with which he was to be associated for most of his future life.

On taking up his new job he lost no time in beginning his study of the actinomycetes and was soon ready to publish an account of his observations, which he did in February 1916. From this work he attained the higher degree of Master of Science but also gained much more than academic distinction, for it led him to formulate certain basic principles, which were to guide him throughout his scientific career to the final triumph of his great discovery. As an undergraduate he had already shown, from his soil sampling of trenches, that bacteria, fungi and actinomycetes differed in their distribution throughout the various depths of soil. The number of bacteria diminished steadily from the surface of the soil downwards, whereas the number of actinomycetes diminished more slowly with increasing depth so that their proportion gradually increased from about 10 per cent on the surface to something like 70 per cent at a depth of 30 inches. He came to the conclusion that micro-organisms live in a somewhat complex community. Some are helpful by providing their neighbours with food but others are destructive, either by consuming those around them, or by otherwise interfering with their growth.

While continuing to observe the distribution of actinomycetes in the soil, he made a careful study of their biochemical and physio-logical activities. During this time, he realized that he rarely came across any disease-producing germs in the soil. This he considered to be very strange, for he was well aware that a large number of organisms infect man, animals and plants, and that these must at some time find their way into the soil, either in excreta or from dead animals. He observed that such organisms tended to disappear rapidly in the soil and asked himself whether it was because they were unable to live in this environment or because they were de-stroyed by other soil microbes. If the latter were true he wondered if soil microbes could be used to combat disease in man. Other people were having similar thoughts and in 1927 Dr Avery of the Rockefeller Institute asked him to recommend a good man trained in soil micro-biology, who could attempt the isolation of an organism from the soil capable of destroying the pneumococcus. Waksman suggested that René Dubos, a young Frenchman who was working in his laboratory at that time, might like to try. By 1932 Dubos managed to isolate a soil bacillus which had the power to destroy the envelope or capsule around the pneumococcus, making it vulnerable to attack by the white cells in the blood stream.

The same year that Dubos made this discovery, Waksman was asked by the National Research Council and the Tuberculosis Association to study the fate of tubercle bacilli in the soil. One of his assistants confirmed, what had in fact been previously shown, that tubercle bacilli do not remain alive for very long there. It was thought that this was possibly because they were attacked by organisms already present in the soil. Waksman therefore encouraged Dubos to study this problem. In 1939, as the result of this investigation, Dubos isolated a substance called tyrothricin from soil bacteria, which had the power to destroy pathogenic organisms. It did not prove to be an ideal therapeutic substance but his discovery was of great import-ance, as it clearly demonstrated to Waksman that this line of research was worthwhile.

Before long Waksman and his team turned once again to the actinomycetes and in 1940, from a culture of one variety of these, they isolated an active substance which they called actinomycin. A detailed study of this substance was now required, but University resources being limited Waksman sought the assistance of Merck, a large pharmaceutical company, and it was with the help of scientists on the staff of this organization that its chemical nature was established and its action in the animal body investigated. This close collaboration between Waksman and his team and members of Merck staff continued for many years, during a time when many antibiotics of importance were isolated and tested, and is an excellent example of how rewarding the partnership between University and industry has so often been in the discovery and development of antibiotics.

Actinomycin proved to be highly toxic to animals and therefore a systematic examination of other actinomycetes and streptomycetes, as well as countless other types of micro-organisms, continued. The work was extremely tedious as it involved not only finding which organisms produced chemical substances, but also the conditions of growth which gave the best yield. It was then necessary to test the inhibitory power of the chemical extracts against various types of organisms, both pathogenic and non-pathogenic. The promising ones had to be purified and concentrated before their toxicity to animals could be assessed. This was followed by a study of their effect on bacteria in animals and, finally, the most promising of them had to be tested against pathogenic organisms in man. This outline of the steps that had to be taken indicates something of the enormity of the task on which Waksman and his team were engaged. They had to face numerous disappointments, but by 1942 they had a measure of success when from a streptomycete they extracted streptothricin. At first this seemed to be promising, showing in the laboratory quite marked activity against organisms not affected by penicillin, but unfortunately although its toxicity was much less than actinomycin it was still too great for clinical use. The search therefore continued and in 1943 their efforts were rewarded when streptomycin was extracted from *Streptomyces griseus*. If is of interest that this organism had first been identified by Waksman and Curtis in 1915 but of course at that time there was no reason why they should have thought of investigating it for antibacterial activity and no suitable tests were devised.

Once the preliminary laboratory studies of Waksman and his

colleagues confirmed the potential importance of streptomycin as an antibiotic, Merck and Company immediately arranged large-scale production of the substance and distributed it free in considerable quantities to a number of hospitals for the purpose of having it tested against the causative organisms of many diseases. It soon became obvious that the discovery was as important as that of penicillin, and further that it was a powerful weapon against many Gram-negative organisms not affected by penicillin, such as those causing urinary tract infections, plague, brucellosis and, above all, tuberculosis. It was fairly quickly superseded by other antibiotics in the treatment of urinary tract infections, but it remains the antibiotic of choice in plague and is still being used in combination with tetracycline against brucellosis. It is, however, in the treatment of tuberculosis that it has made, and is continuing to make, its most important contribution.

Waksman lost no time early in 1944 in exposing tubercle bacilli on culture plates to streptomycin and soon found that their growth was markedly inhibited. Soon after announcing this exciting observation, he was approached by Dr Feldman and Dr. Hinshaw, of the Mayo Clinic in Rochester, Minnesota, requesting permission to test the effectiveness of streptomycin in guinea-pigs infected with tuberculosis. Their initial experiments with small amounts of the substance were so promising that Merck and Company then supplied them with larger amounts of the material, and in 1945 the use of this in humans fully confirmed the results of their animal experiments. Physicians with special experience of tuberculosis, both in America and Great Britain, quickly became extremely interested, with the result that for the first time in medical history large-scale, statistically controlled clinical trials were undertaken, all of which demonstrated the out-standing importance of this antibiotic in the fight against a disease which has been a scourge of man for centuries.

9

THE WHITE PLAGUE

Tuberculosis has been one of man's main enemies for centuries and, although a certain amount of control was achieved by improved hygiene, sanitation and housing in some parts of the world during the earlier part of this century, there was no hope of successfully conquering it until the introduction of effective chemotherapy after the Second World War. Previously treatment usually gave only temporary benefit so that the disease often recurred and ultimately proved fatal. Due to the use of potent drugs during recent years, the mortality rate has been falling rapidly in most highly developed countries although the disease is still widespread in those parts of the world where the drugs are scarce or badly used.

The discovery of streptomycin and its powerful effect against the tubercle bacillus was a great therapeutic advance, but it was soon realized that it was of very limited value when used by itself. When first given to a patient the effect on the disease was remarkable: the patient's general condition rapidly improved, and X-rays of the lungs showed surprisingly rapid clearing of abnormal shadows. But after some weeks, it was found that it began to lose its effect and finally became useless. The reason for this is that tubercle bacilli in some way adapt themselves to streptomycin and become resistant to its action, so that they are no longer killed, but continue to multiply in its presence. This development by bacteria of what is called 'drug resistance' is not confined to the action of streptomycin on tubercle bacilli, but also occurs with many other antibiotics in their action on other organisms. This big problem is seriously affecting man's conquest of many bacterial diseases, but in the case of tuberculosis a way to overcome the difficulty with streptomycin has fortunately been discovered.

While Waksman was at work on soil microbes, other scientists were experimenting with various chemical substances, and testing them, by a method of trial and error, against the tubercle bacillus. Usually there was no clue as to which might prove effective, so that the work was laborious and time-consuming. In 1941 Bernheim gave a definite lead when he noted that salicylates suppressed the growth of tubercle bacilli on laboratory culture plates, by interfering with their oxygenation. Lehmann in Sweden followed up Bernheim's clue by testing a large number of different salicylic acid compounds against tubercle bacilli in the laboratory and found that *para*-aminosalicylic acid (P.A.S.) was the most promising. Next he administered it to guinea-pigs and rats to check for any toxic reactions and finally considered it was safe to give it to patients.

In March 1944 twenty tuberculous patients in Gothenburg were given the drug. It was reported that their general condition improved, with reduction of fever, increased appetite and gain in weight. It was soon found however that by itself its effect on tuberculosis in man was not as good as had been initially supposed, and at one stage it looked as if its use might be abandoned. Fortunately, as it was discovered about the same time as streptomycin, it was not long before the two drugs were used in combination. To everyone's surprise, it was found that when the two were given together, streptomycin no longer lost its effect after a short time because of the development of bacterial resistance, but could be profitably administered for many months. This was probably the most important step in the battle against tuberculosis. Much work had still to be done to determine the optimum dosage for these two drugs and the length of time for which they should be given. It was found that if the daily dose was too big there were serious toxic side effects, but that it was necessary to continue treatment for many months in order to avoid relapse.

Until then, when any new drug had been discovered, separate small trials had been carried out by individual physicians on a limited number of patients, which meant that no one could gain more than a clinical impression as to the efficacy of the substance. Initial pilot studies to assess the value of streptomycin against tuberculosis were done at the Mayo Clinic in America, and the results published in 1944. Following this, however, and for the first time in medical history, large scientifically controlled trials were organized in Great Britain by the Medical Research Council in co-operation with the

Research Committee of the British Tuberculosis Association, and in America by the Veterans Administration, the United States Public Health Service and, in the early phase, by the American Trudeau Society. Hundreds of patients with widespread, rapidly progressive tuberculosis of the lungs were admitted into these trials. Half were given the standard orthodox treatment of that time, and the other half were given the new drugs. The progress of the two groups was then compared, both by clinical examination and radiological assessment, and in this way it was possible to measure exactly and quickly the advantages and any disadvantages, of these new drugs. At the same time, by dividing the main groups into sub-groups, a comparison could be made as to the efficacy of various treatment regimes, the optimum dosage and duration of treatment.

The result of the first trial in this country using streptomycin by itself was published jointly by the Medical Research Council and the British Tuberculosis Association in 1948. Following this, similar controlled trials were carried out using *para*-aminosalicylic acid (P.A.S.) alone and also using the two drugs simultaneously. The final results were published in November 1950, but at the end of 1949 the enormous advantages of using the two drugs together in the prevention of streptomycin resistance became obvious. It was not felt justifiable therefore to withhold this information until the trial had been formally completed, so an interim communication was published in the British medical press in December 1949, and a similar report, by American workers, was published in the American Review of Tuberculosis in the same year. This was the most important observation ever made in the treatment of tuberculosis, and a turning point in the history of man's fight against the disease. It still meant that patients needed many months of treatment, but it enabled streptomycin to assert its powerful effect over long periods, and thus gradually but surely to kill the millions of tubercle bacilli living and dividing in diseased tissue.

At the same time as these drugs were being used in hospital wards, work was going on in the laboratory to find other drugs which might prove to be even better. After Domagk discovered Prontosil, a large number of sulphonamide drugs were produced and tested systematically against the tubercle bacillus. None proved to be particularly powerful, but one or two showed sufficient promise to lead Domagk to examine other chemical substances with similar structures. In this way, twelve years after his original discovery of Prontosil, he was able to show that an entirely new group of substances, the thiosemicarbazones, had a marked inhibitory effect on the tubercle bacillus in the laboratory. Although they were not to prove of great value in the treatment of tuberculosis, they nevertheless were of great importance, because it was from a systematic study of them that scientists were eventually led to examine the effect of various derivatives of nicotinic acid. One of these, isonicotinic acid hydrazide (isoniazid) was to prove outstandingly useful.

Isonicotinic acid hydrazide had been synthesized in the laboratory by Hans Meyer and Josef Mally as long ago as 1912, at a time when people were willing to believe in anti-microbial therapy following the introduction of arsphenamine by Ehrlich less than two years previously, but unfortunately no one was then looking for an anti-tuberculous drug. On the other hand, by the middle of this century, in the light of success already attained, many research centres were actively looking for anti-tuberculous compounds. By 1951 three independent pharmaceutical firms, Hoffmann la Roche, Squibb and Bayer, knowing nothing of each other's work, had undertaken a study of isomers of nicotinic acid, as a direct result of systematic work on the thiosemicarbazone group. Each firm separately concluded that isoniazid showed such promise that it must be tried out on human beings, so they approached three different clinical centres; Hoffmann la Roche went to Drs Robitsek and Selikoff at the Seaview Hospital, Staten Island, New York; Squibb approached Professor Walsh McDermott at Cornell University; and Bayer went to Professor Klee at Elberfeld. A situation therefore arose whereby three medical centres were conducting clinical trials on the same drug, each one unaware that there were others doing similar work. Professor McDermott has described an amusing incident which occurred when Gerard Domagk visited his laboratory on 28 September 1951. Considerable discussion took place on the subject of anti-tuberculous drugs in general, and the thiosemicarbazones in particular. Neither however mentioned that he was taking part in a clinical trial of isoniazid, and in retrospect McDermott feels certain that each one must have walked away from their meeting with the thought, 'Isn't he in for a surprise'. In fact they were both to have a big surprise because neither knew of the existence of the Hoffmann la Roche clinical trial which Drs Robitsek and Selikoff had already started. Nevertheless, the three groups came eventually together, and arrangements were made for publication of the results in scientific journals in the first week of April 1952. Unfortunately a highly dramatized and sensational account exploded in the lay press some time before this, telling the world that at last a miracle cure had been discovered for tuberculosis. As a result sufferers all over the world began to demand this drug before it had been properly assessed. A leading article in *The Lancet* on 5 April 1952, drawing attention to this, stated that it was most unfortunate that such sensational statements had been made, because, as the drug could be produced cheaply in large quantities and was easy to take, it would be a great temptation for physicians to prescribe it for all tuberculous patients, whether in hospital, or at home without adequate supervision or safeguards. It pointed out that in America general distribution had not yet been authorized, and it hoped that the profession in this country would be no less careful. It stated that there were very real risks in the widespread and uncontrolled use of drugs before they have been properly evaluated, particularly in the case of this drug, as it was not yet known whether drug resistance would develop, as had happened with streptomycin. In the summer the Ministry of Health also issued a similar statement. In spite of these warnings, the drug was given by itself to thousands of tuberculous patients, and in every case the tubercle bacilli became resistant to the drug so that it ceased to be effective after a few weeks. The results of clinical trials showed that it retained its power for very long periods, providing it was prescribed with either streptomycin or para-aminosalicylic acid.

It has therefore become an established practice always to prescribe these drugs in combination, either in pairs or sometimes all three together. Further, it has been found essential to continue daily treatment for about two years in the majority of cases. Unfortunately, it has been found difficult to persuade certain people to take the drugs regularly, and in the prescribed combination. The result is similar to taking one drug by itself, with the development of tubercle bacilli resistant to the drugs, so that not only does their disease become untreatable, but also other people are liable to be infected with these dangerous organisms. This problem is particularly common in many underdeveloped countries, where it is seriously impeding the eradication of the disease.

The disadvantages associated with streptomycin having to be administered by repeated injection, and with P.A.S. causing much nausea and at times diarrhoea, coupled with the fact that an increasing number of strains of tubercle bacilli have been developing resistance to these two drugs and to isoniazid, either singly or in combination, have led over the years to a systematic search for other suitable drugs. Capreomycin, cycloserine, ethionamide, kanamycin, pyrazinamide and viomycin all have a varying amount of activity against the tubercle bacillus, but as they all have considerable toxicity they are only employed when bacterial resistance has rendered the original three drugs useless.

Ethambutol, a synthetic compound which when tested in 1961 by J. P. Thomas and his colleagues in America was found to be effective in experimental tuberculous infection in mice, is one substance which is being increasingly used as a drug of first choice. It is, however, the discovery of rifampicin which has been the most outstanding advance in the treatment of tuberculosis since the discovery of streptomycin and isoniazid. The rifamycins are a group of antibiotics isolated from *Streptomyces mediterranei* and studied in the laboratories of Lepetit in Milan during the 1960's. Rifampicin, the most outstanding of 500 synthetic derivatives of one of these rifamycins, was painstakingly produced by Ciba of Basle and Lepetit working in collaboration. It is active against many bacteria but much the most important use of this drug is in the fight against tuberculosis. Its ready absorption when taken by mouth gives it a great advantage over streptomycin and its anti-tuberculous activity being equal to that of isoniazid makes these two in combination extremely effective in the treatment of this disease.

10

A MICROBE FROM THE SEA

In 1945, at a time when penicillin was already being extensively employed and streptomycin was just coming into use, Giuseppe Brotzu, Professor of Bacteriology at Cagliari University in Sardinia, made an observation which was eventually to lead to the development of yet another important group of antibiotics, the cephalosporins.

Brotzu was a politician and administrator in addition to being a bacteriologist, but in spite of his many activities he decided to investigate the interesting phenomenon that the sea around the coast at Cagliari, where sewage was discharged into it from the town, was remarkably free from disease-producing bacteria. It was no doubt discoveries such as those already made by Fleming and Waksman that led him to wonder whether this might be because bacteria were being destroyed by some other micro-organism, so in 1948 with this in mind he examined the area and was justly rewarded by recovering from the sea near the sewage outfall a mould known as *Cephalosporium acremonium*. He lost no time in making a crude extract from this mould and administering it to patients with various infections, including staphylococcal abscesses, typhoid fever and brucellosis. Although there must have been remarkably little antibiotic material in his extract, the treatment appears to have been sufficiently successful for him to realize that he had made a discovery of importance. He therefore knew that the next step must be to obtain the active principle in pure form, but feeling that he was not capable of doing this himself he turned for assistance to the Italian pharmaceutical industry. Finding no help from that source he decided in 1948 to publish his findings with the express hope that others with greater facilities than himself would read the report and continue his work. It is somewhat surprising that Professor Domenico Marotta, the Director of the Italian Institute of Public Health in Rome, did not show any interest, because by that time he had a special department of chemical microbiology and it was in 1948 that he invited

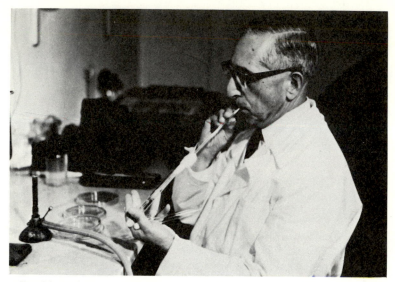

Fig. 54. *Professor Giuseppe Brotzu at his laboratory in Cagliari, Sardinia.*

Ernst Chain to take charge of it. Brotzu's report of his discovery was very nearly overlooked, because instead of inserting it in some internationally read journal he placed it in a private publication entitled 'On the Works of The Institute of Hygiene of Cagliari'. Fortunately he sent a copy to Dr Blyth Brook, whom he had known when the latter was a British Public Health Officer in Sardinia, in the hope that he might be able to interest someone in England in his discovery. Blyth Brook consulted the British Medical Research Council who in turn referred him to Sir Howard Florey at Oxford. Florey immediately showed interest in the discovery and asked Brotzu to send a copy of his paper, together with a sample of his mould, to Oxford, so that two members of his team, E. P. Abraham (Fig. 47, p. 117) and G. G. F. Newton, could pursue the matter further. Abraham, who is now Professor of Chemical Pathology at Oxford, had already by that time had much experience in antibiotic research having worked closely with Florey, Chain and others in investigating the penicillium mould and therefore he and Newton were delighted to take up this further challenge. It was to result in many years of work, which although at times was frustrating,

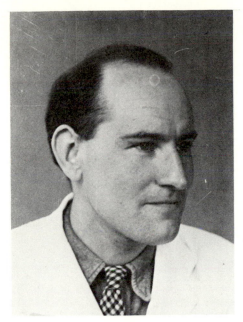

Fig. 55. Dr G. G. F. Newton (1920–69).

eventually proved to be very rewarding and it is sad to relate that in 1969, just at a time when the cephalosporins were at last finding an established place in clinical medicine, Dr Newton died from a coronary thrombosis at the relatively young age of forty-nine.

Abraham assumed that the journal they received from Sardinia was published regularly and it was only some years later when he met Brotzu that he discovered that it was a unique issue which Brotzu said was only to appear again if and when anything of comparable importance was discovered!

The fact that Brotzu had found his antibiotic extract was active against such diverse organisms as staphylococci and typhoid bacilli meant that it had a broad spectrum of activity against both Gram-positive and Gram-negative organisms and therefore Abraham and Newton were very puzzled when they first extracted from the culture fluid a substance which was only active against Gram-positive organisms. They therefore re-examined the culture fluid and found that there was a second substance present which was active against

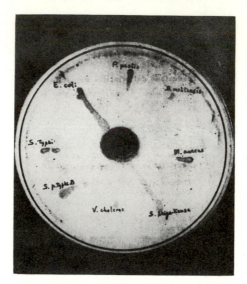

Fig. 56. Brotzu's original culture plate (1948) showing inhibition of growth of many bacteria due to the action of the cephalosporium mould.

Gram-negative organisms. They therefore called the first substance cephalosporin P, an antibiotic which has since turned out to have a structure very similar to fusidic acid, a powerful anti-staphylococcal agent isolated from a strain of *Fusidium coccineum* in 1962, and the second one cephalosporin N, which as it has subsequently been shown to have the chemical structure of a penicillin, is now often referred to as penicillin N. This substance has been used in small-scale clinical trials under the name of adicillin, with success in typhoid fever, but up to now it has not become available on a commercial basis and the cephalosporins might well by now have been forgotten had it not been that in 1953 Abraham and Newton, during the course of a purely academic study of cephalosporin N (penicillin N) stumbled by chance on yet a third cephalosporin which they named cephalosporin C. They immediately appreciated that this was an extremely promising substance, because not only did it show evidence of activity against both Gram-positive and Gram-negative organisms, but above all it showed evidence of resistance to the penicillinase secreted by certain strains of staphylococci. This invoked

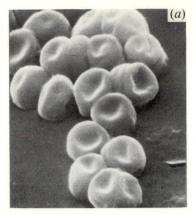
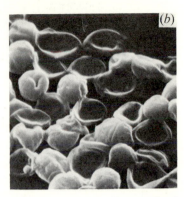

Fig. 57(a). An electron micrograph of Staphylococcus aureus *after one hour's exposure to fusidic acid, an antibiotic with a chemical structure similar to that of cephalosporin P.* (b) Staphylococcus aureus *three hours after exposure to fusidic acid.*

much excitement, as by that time penicillinase-producing staphylococci resistant to penicillin were becoming an increasing menace in all hospitals, and methicillin, the first semi-synthetic penicillin capable of combating this organism, had not yet been discovered. This property of cephalosporin C alone therefore made it worthy of very close attention, but the production of it in sufficient quantities for clinical trials from the original Sardinian cephalosporium mould proved extremely difficult and Abraham therefore sought the assistance of scientists at the Medical Research Council's Antibiotic Research Station at Clevedon, near Bristol.

The patent for cephalosporin C in accordance with the Medical Research Council's policy at that time had been assigned to the National Research Development Corporation (N.R.D.C.). This organization, set up by the British government under an Act of Parliament in 1949 for the purpose of protecting, developing and exploiting inventions in the public interest, was to play an important part in controlling and co-ordinating the many groups of workers who eventually were to make important contributions in this particular field of study. When the N.R.D.C. initially invited British pharmaceutical companies with fermentation facilities to assist in the production of cephalosporin C, only Glaxo showed any real interest.

Accordingly in 1956 the Corporation organized meetings between this company's scientists and workers both at Oxford and Clevedon. The following year the Clevedon group made an important advance when they isolated a mutant of the Sardinian organism, No. 8650, which yielded much larger amounts of cephalosporin C than could be obtained from the parent strain. It was from this mutant that Glaxo Laboratories then produced 100 grams of the substance, which was more than sufficient for Abraham and Newton in 1959 to confirm its chemical structure and for Florey to demonstrate its extremely low toxicity when injected into mice and to show that it was able to protect these animals from infection with penicillinase-producing strains of staphylococci not responsive to treatment with penicillin.

Cephalosporin C's antibacterial activity had always been known to be weak, but in view of Florey's successful animal experiments it was planned to give very large amounts of it by intravenous drip to patients with penicillin-resistant staphylococcal infections. But before this could be done Beecham Research Laboratories discovered methicillin. It therefore became apparent that, if the work already done on the Sardinian mould was not to be wasted, it was essential for the nucleus of the cephalosporin C molecule to be identified so that it could be used as the basic structure around which more potent cephalosporin substances could be built. Abraham and Newton found it a relatively straightforward task to remove the alpha-aminoadipyl side chain from cephalosporin C and by this manoeuvre, by July 1959, obtained minute amounts of the substance's nucleus, which on analysis proved to be 7-aminocephalosporanic acid (7-ACA). What they found very difficult however was to produce 7-ACA in quantity.

Many pharmaceutical companies in addition to Glaxo had by 1960 applied to the National Research Development Corporation for permission to work with cephalosporin C. These included the American firms Eli Lilly, Merck and Company, Charles Pfizer and Company and Smith Kline and French; as well as Ciba in Switzerland, Farmitalia in Italy and, by 1961, the Fujisawa Pharmaceutical Company in Japan.

In searching for a method for producing 7-ACA in bulk from cephalosporin C all concerned were looking for an enzyme capable of removing the alpha-aminoadipyl side chain, but extensive searches by these pharmaceutical companies failed to discover it. This was a period of considerable disappointment, but just at the time when it looked as if no further progress could be made the situation was transformed by Eli Lilly Research Laboratories discovering, towards the end of 1960, an ingenious chemical procedure which enabled an appreciable quantity of the nucleus to be obtained from cephalosporin C. By this time both Eli Lilly and Glaxo could produce large amounts of the latter by fermentation, so there was now no difficulty in obtaining as much 7-ACA as required. It then became a matter of systematically adding various side chains to this nucleus and patiently testing the various substances produced to see which of them was likely to be of use in medicine. It was Eli Lilly who had the first success when, by adding a thienyl acetyl group to the cephalosporin nucleus, they produced cephalothin, a powerful antibiotic with a wide range of antibacterial activity. This first cephalosporin was not absorbed when taken by mouth and when given by intramuscular injection was extremely painful, but fortunately Glaxo soon after marketed another preparation, cephaloridine, which though it has to be injected is far less unpleasant and still widely used. The search then continued for a cephalosporin which could be given by mouth. The first appeared in 1961 under the name of cephaloglycin but this was poorly absorbed and has since been replaced by both Eli Lilly and Glaxo producing cephalexin. Several other cephalosporins have since been manufactured, including one marketed independently by E. R. Squibb and Smith Kline and French, known as cephradine. This antibiotic has the distinction of being the only one of this group which can be either given by injection or taken by mouth.

There are therefore now available a number of different cephalosporins, each having much the same range of antibacterial activity and capable of killing both Gram-positive organisms, including penicillinase-producing staphylococci, and many of the commoner Gram-negative ones, so that in broad terms any one cephalosporin has an effectiveness equivalent to the sum total of penicillin G, penicillin V, ampicillin and flucloxacillin. In practice, of the two groups of antibiotics, the penicillins are far more commonly prescribed. This is partly because the cephalosporins are still rather

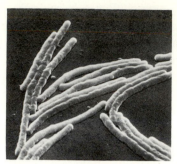

Fig. 58. An electron micrograph of Escherichia coli *elongated and deformed after exposure to the oral cephalosporin, cephalexin.*

more expensive as a result of the high cost of their initial development but also because the various penicillins were firmly established in clinical practice before the cephalosporins became available. It is interesting to contemplate whether the medical profession's prescribing habits over the years might not have been somewhat different if it had been the cephalosporin nucleus rather than the penicillin nucleus which had been the first to be discovered. Such speculation apart, there can be no doubt that the successful conclusion to the cephalosporin story after many years of diligent research was the result of a combination of good fortune and dogged determination. It was eight years between the isolation of the cephalosporium mould in Sardinia and the discovery of cephalosporin C in Oxford, and even then the latter was only a chance finding during the course of an academic experiment. It was then a further seven years before this substance's nucleus could be produced in sufficient quantity to permit the construction of a number of important antibiotic substances. It was in referring to this latter very worrying time that E. P. Abraham and P. B. Loder, writing in a book *Cephalosporins and Penicillins* published in 1972, said 'the difficulties to be overcome appeared at times to be so formidable that it would not have been surprising if the project had been abandoned. Its final success must be attributed to a combination of scientific ability, technical expertise, and willingness to take calculated risks in the pharmaceutical companies that were mainly involved'.

11

MORE MICROBES FROM THE SOIL

The successful extraction of penicillin from the airborne mould *Penicillium notatum* and streptomycin from the soil microbe *Streptomyces griseus*, led to a systematic search throughout the world for other micro-organisms with antibacterial activity. Over the years there can scarcely have been a single mould or similar micro-organism which has not been subjected to scrutiny. For example, in 1945 even the mould which grew on the isinglass covering the photograph of a bacteriologist's wife did not escape inspection! The bacteriologist was the American R. E. Shope and the place was the Pacific Island of Guam where he was stationed at that time. The mould turned out to be a strain of *Penicillium funiculosum*, from which he ultimately managed to extract an antibiotic which has proved to have a certain amount of antiviral activity. He called this antibiotic helenine, explaining that he chose this name partly because it was non-descriptive, non-committal and not pre-empted but 'largely out of recognition of the good taste shown by the mold...in locating on the picture of my wife!'

Then there was the pink mould-like substance which in 1947 drew attention to itself by having the temerity to grow on a damp wall inside a bacteriologist's Parisian house. The bacteriologist, L. J. Decaris, found this to be a strain of *Streptomyces lavendulae* from which the pharmaceutical company Roussel eventually extracted the antibiotic framycetin.

Since then it has been from various other streptomycetes that many important antibiotics have been extracted. The first major breakthrough came in 1947 when J. Ehrlich and his colleagues found a streptomycete in soil in Venezuela, and H. E. Carter and others found a similar organism in a sample of soil taken from a compost heap in Illinois, from both of which the two groups independently extracted the antibiotic chloramphenicol. Since then it has proved possible to manufacture this antibiotic by a synthetic process, a method of production which is unique amongst clinically important antibiotics.

The next outstanding advance was the discovery of a group of antibiotics now known collectively as the tetracyclines. The first produced by the Lederle Laboratories Division of the American Cyanamid Company was Aureomycin. This antibiotic was extracted in 1948 from *Streptomyces aureofaciens*, which was given this name because of the yellow colour of its colonies; this was followed two years later by Charles Pfizer and Company producing Terramycin, a substance derived from *Streptomyces rimosus*. Subsequent analysis showed that chemically they were almost identical and accordingly they were given the official names of chlortetracycline and oxytetracycline respectively.

In 1953 a third member of the group, known as tetracycline, was introduced. Structurally simpler and yet clinically as effective as the other two this antibiotic is obtainable either by extraction from a *Streptomyces* or by chemical modification of chlortetracycline. In subsequent years many other 'tetracyclines' have appeared, some capable of being given by injection and all better absorbed when given by mouth than the original three.

When chloramphenicol and the tetracyclines were first introduced around the beginning of the 1950's they had certain apparent advantages over the other two antibiotics available at that time, namely penicillin and streptomycin. Both penicillin and streptomycin have to be given by injection and both individually have a limited range of antibacterial activity, with penicillin being mainly effective against Gram-positive organisms and streptomycin against Gram-negative ones, whereas chloramphenicol and the tetracyclines may be given by mouth and initially each one was effective against a very wide range of bacteria both Gram-positive and Gram-negative. It was in describing this remarkable breadth of activity of these substances that the term 'broad spectrum' was introduced into the medical language. One of their big disadvantages however is that their action, which is merely to slow down the speed of reproduction of bacteria, a process known as bacteriostasis, is dependent on cells forming part of the body's defence system for finally destroying the organisms. This is in contrast to penicillin, streptomycin and various other antibiotics since introduced, such as ampicillin and the cephalosporins, which have a direct killing or bactericidal effect on bacteria.

Chloramphenicol quickly won considerable acclaim when late in 1947 the small amount available at that time was used with considerable success in controlling an outbreak of typhus fever in Bolivia. It also soon proved to be remarkably effective against the *Salmonella* organisms responsible for typhoid and paratyphoid fever. It was however its broad spectrum activity against the commonly occurring Gram-positive organisms, such as staphylococci, streptococci and pneumococci, and the Gram-negative ones, such as *Haemophilus influenzae* and *Escherichia coli*, which rapidly led to it being extensively used in the treatment of many of the more mundane type of infections affecting both children and adults.

Unfortunately by 1950, despite the fact that it had passed stringent toxicity tests in animals, there was evidence that occasionally it is capable of causing serious and at times fatal damage to the bone marrow with destruction of the red and white blood cell precursors. Initially reports of this were sporadic and passed almost unnoticed, but during the course of the next two years they appeared too frequently to be ignored and by 1963 the Registry of Blood Dyscrasias of the American Medical Association had collected statistics proving that the antibiotic was responsible for more cases of bone marrow damage than all other drugs put together. Although the exact incidence of this is difficult to assess because the total number of people subject to this risk is not known, the disturbing feature is that it is an idiosyncratic response which occurs unpredictably and after exposure to the smallest possible dose. It is for this reason, and also because of somewhat complex problems associated with bacterial resistance which will be fully discussed in the next chapter, that most physicians consider that the antibiotic should no longer be used in the treatment of routine infections but reserved for combating typhoid and paratyphoid fever against which, in spite of its side effects, it is still the drug of choice.

From the time the tetracyclines were first introduced in the early 1950's, because of their broad spectrum range of activity against a considerable number of Gram-positive and Gram-negative organisms, their ready absorption into the body when taken by mouth and their relative freedom from side effects, they remained extremely popular in the treatment of many commonly occurring infections for the next ten to fifteen years.

The side effects initially reported were mainly gastro-intestinal, but after many years of use other complications were recognized, including disfiguring staining of teeth in young children, renal failure in those with previously damaged kidneys, and the occasional curious increase in cerebrospinal fluid pressure, mainly in infants.

The tetracyclines were for many years widely used in the treatment of streptococcal sore throats and pneumococcal pneumonia but by the middle of the 1960's the emergence of many resistant strains of *Streptococcus pyogenes* and pneumococci precluded their further use in these infections. They were also much employed in the suppression of *Haemophilus influenzae* occurring in acute exacerbations of chronic bronchitis, until at about the same time the more effective bactericidal antibiotic ampicillin was introduced. An increase in resistance amongst Gram-negative enterobacteria, such as *Escherichia coli*, has also led to a decline in their use in urinary tract infections.

One or other of the tetracycline group is still the treatment of choice in the particular form of pneumonia caused by the *Mycoplasma pneumoniae*, also in the treatment of non-specific urethritis and may be used as an alternative in the treatment of gonorrhoea and syphilis in those allergic to penicillin. This group of antibiotics is also useful in the treatment of typhus fever and cholera. They have also been advocated in the treatment of the eye infection trachoma, but the results are disappointing.

Erythromycin, an antibiotic obtained in 1952 by the Lilly Research Laboratories in Indianapolis from a strain of *Streptomyces erythreus* found in soil from the Philippines, was widely used for many years in combating commonly occurring Gram-positive organisms. Its discovery in the early 1950's was particularly fortuitous as it had a powerful effect on the increasing number of staphylococci which by that time had developed resistance to penicillin. Unfortunately staphylococcal resistance to this antibiotic also occurred fairly rapidly, but nevertheless it played an important part in combating this organism until the more powerful semi-synthetic penicillin, methicillin, was introduced in the early 1960's. It continued to be used against pneumococci and streptococci but by 1968 a certain amount of resistance to these organisms was also reported

Lincomycin is another antibiotic which closely resembles erythromycin in its activity against Gram-positive organisms, including staphylococci, streptococci and pneumococci. This antibiotic, discovered in 1962 in the laboratories of the Upjohn Company, was given this name because it was obtained from a previously undescribed streptomycete found in soil in Lincoln, Nebraska and therefore subsequently named *Streptomyces lincolnensis*. The antibiotic's remarkable ability to penetrate bone made it particularly useful in the treatment of acute staphylococcal osteomyelitis, but since 1967 it has been replaced by a synthetic modification known as clindamycin, an antibiotic with the same range of activity but which is many times more powerful than the parent substance.

Finally there are four important bactericidal antibiotics which share with streptomycin a similar chemical structure, non-absorption when taken by mouth and a tendency to cause either giddiness or deafness when injected into the body. These include framycetin, the discovery of which has already been discussed; neomycin, first isolated by Waksman and Lechevalier in 1949 from a strain of *Streptomyces fradiae* found in New Jersey soil; kanamycin, isolated in 1957 by Umezawa and others from *Streptomyces kanamyceticus* which they found in soil in Japan; and, in addition, gentamicin. This is spelt with an 'i' because the suffix 'mycin' has come to imply derivation from a *Streptomyces*, whereas this antibiotic, discovered in 1963, is a product of a strain of *Micromonospora purpurea*.

Framycetin and neomycin are very similar and because of their toxic effects are rarely injected into the body, but mainly used for external application to the skin and for oral use in order to suppress the normal flora of the bowel as part of the treatment of acute liver failure and sometimes before operations on the gut. Kanamycin may also be given by mouth for this purpose, or it may be given by injection in the treatment of certain intractable urinary tract infections. The most important of the group however is gentamicin because this powerful antibiotic, when given by injection, is of great use in treating severe staphylococcal infections and in combating the life-threatening septicaemia which may occur as a result of infection with various Gram-negative enterobacteria.

This completes the review of the discovery of some of the more important antimicrobial substances. It is hoped that from this it will be seen that advances have not come solely from chance observations by able men with prepared minds, but have required in addition much systematic work by teams of academic scientists working in close co-operation with colleagues in highly competitive pharmaceutical companies who, being free from the dead hand of monopolistic State control, have been willing to invest enormous sums of money in research projects without any guarantee of ultimate profit. It was an awareness of the importance of free enterprise in medical research that led Abraham in lecturing to an American audience in 1974 to say 'in these days, in which governments are showing signs of restricting their grants for research more and more to those which they think may pay off in the near future, this is perhaps an argument for allowing some of our resources to be used to satisfy the long-term curiosity of scientists without requiring an immediate return' and for Chain, at the first joint meeting of the Royal College of Physicians of London and the Royal Society three years earlier, to remark even more forcibly

If one considers the immense effort that was expended in the search for new antibiotics of clinical usefulness, the result must be considered as meagre. Many hundreds of people participated in the effort, and hundreds of millions of dollars were spent on screening micro-organisms from the air, the earth and water with the result of a dozen or so antibiotics of clinical importance. The effort was possible only because it was distributed over a large number of independent groups that shared the risk. No centrally organised state organisation would have been able to sponsor such effort. One could not imagine the civil servant who would have had the courage to spend such very large sums of money on a project that could not be guaranteed to be successful. These simple facts should not be forgotten in discussions on the desirability of nationalising the pharmaceutical industry.

The medical profession is certainly very well aware that it relies heavily on commercial firms continuing to invest enormous sums of money in intensive research aimed at providing new antimicrobial substances to replace those no longer of use because of the development of bacterial resistance. The various methods employed by bacteria in defending themselves against attack by antibiotics will now be discussed.

12

ENEMY RESISTANCE

Man's discovery of antimicrobial agents must surely rank as one of his greatest triumphs. The introduction into medical practice of the sulphonamides in the 1930's, penicillin and streptomycin in the 1940's, the broad spectrum bacteriostatic antibiotics during the 1950's, the broad spectrum bactericidal ones in the 1960's, together with other important synthetic chemicals and highly specific narrow spectrum antibiotics during these years, have all been outstanding achievements revolutionizing the treatment of bacterial disease.

It is essential however that no one should underestimate the cunning of bacteria, who with remarkable ingenuity have developed methods of resisting the action of these substances so that some have already been rendered useless, whilst others are in great danger of it. This defensive action by bacteria, which for the sake of brevity is often referred to as drug resistance, will therefore be discussed in detail.

Some bacteria which are initially sensitive to an antibiotic achieve resistance to it by the evolution of mutant strains which, because of subtle changes either in their structure or biochemistry, are capable of blocking its action. Other bacteria during the course of their long evolutionary history have learned to protect themselves from some of the higher forms of microbial life by developing enzymes which are harmful to them and consequently, because of their ability to secrete these chemical substances, are now able to destroy some of the antibiotics which man in recent years has extracted from these more advanced types of micro-organisms.

A number of bacteria carry much of their information concerning resistance locked up in their chromosomes and therefore are able to pass this on from generation to generation during the course of reproduction by binary fission. Others carry similar knowledge in plasmids. These structures consisting of small pieces of gene-containing deoxyribonucleic acid (DNA) are separate from the chromosomes.

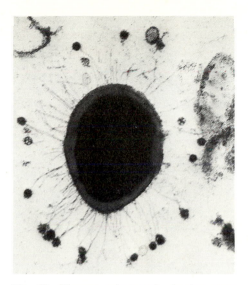

Fig. 59. Electron micrograph showing many bacteriophages attached to a staphylococcus, some with their heads filled with DNA, others with them empty having transferred this material into the bacterial cell, a process which is necessary for the reproduction of these viruses inside the bacterial cell but at the same time enabling genetic information concerning antibiotic resistance to be transferred from one staphylococcus to another.

This extrachromosomal genetic material is not only replicated in every newly produced bacterial cell, but what is so remarkable is that bacteria have devised means whereby they can transmit this material from one mature bacterial cell to another. This is done either, as in the case of staphylococci, by employing viruses known as bacteriophages (see also Figs. 24 and 25) as carriers in the process known as transduction (see p. 43). or, in the case of certain Gram-negative bacilli, by pairs of organisms undergoing an act of conjugation resembling that employed by more highly developed animal species for sexual reproduction.

Penicillin is the one antibiotic to which no initially sensitive organism, with the exception of the gonococcus, has ever managed to develop resistance. This means that *Streptococcus pyogenes*, the

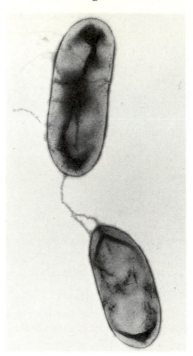

Fig. 60. Two Escherichia coli
undergoing conjugation.

pneumococcus and the spirochaete of syphilis, in common with
many other organisms, are still as readily killed by this substance as
they were when it was first introduced in the early 1940's. The same
applies to all initially sensitive staphylococci. The reason why
staphylococci are now becoming increasingly resistant to penicillin
is not because sensitive strains have acquired resistance, but because
when the antibiotic was introduced there were already a few strains
possessing natural resistance to it, and the gradual destruction of most
of the sensitive ones over the years has encouraged their proliferation.
The gonococcus is the only organism which over the years has
gradually acquired increasing resistance to this antibiotic. It is partly
because of this, but also because the permissiveness of modern
society is encouraging its spread, that gonorrhoea, a disease which
just after World War II appeared to be coming under control, has

once again reached epidemic proportions in most big cities of the world.

Experience with all other anti-microbial agents introduced during the past forty years has been that bacteria sooner or later start to develop resistance to them, but that the facility with which this happens is widely variable and depends on the antibiotic and the organism concerned.

The manner in which bacterial resistance to an antibiotic may steadily increase once it has been widely used for some time in the community is well illustrated by the response of *Streptococcus pyogenes* to the action of tetracycline. When this antibiotic was first introduced in the early 1950's all strains of this organism were uniformly sensitive to it. After about a year a few resistant ones started to emerge and although by 1958 these still only comprised less than 1 per cent of the streptococcal population, by 1965 the number had risen to 44 per cent. Such a high percentage of resistant strains meant that the antibiotic could no longer be used against this particular organism with any measure of confidence. It is interesting that the consequent decrease in the use of this antibiotic has been associated with the proportion of resistant strains dropping to 27 per cent by 1971. Events such as this have led to the realization that when a particular organism starts to develop appreciable numbers of resistant strains to an antibiotic it is often better temporarily to withdraw the latter and to use alternatives in rotation rather than to run the risk of allowing it to become prematurely obsolescent.

The development of resistance to antibiotics in regular use in the community has until recently never been a matter for particular concern, because in general this has taken place slowly and by the time one anti-microbial agent has become ineffectual there have always been others to take its place. The situation inside hospitals has however always been rather different, because in such a closed environment the high concentration of bacteria, the large quantities of antibiotics used, and the ease with which cross infection can occur, are all factors which encourage the rapid development of drug resistance and it is in these institutions that resistant staphylococci and enterobacteria are proving to be particularly troublesome.

Staphylococcus aureus is widely distributed throughout the community, frequently living as a commensal on the skin and in the nose, but is also the cause of many different types of serious infection (p. 34). The powerful destructive effect of penicillin on staphylococci when this antibiotic was first brought into clinical use in 1940, and the miraculous manner in which it was responsible for saving the lives of patients dying from uncontrolled infection with this organism, was so dramatic as to remain vividly in the memory of all those of us who witnessed it. It was therefore a cause for much concern when Mary Barber, a few years later, reported a rapidly increasing incidence of strains resistant to penicillin in hospitals. The frequency of these was 14 per cent, 38 per cent and 59 per cent in the years 1946 to 1948 respectively, and by 1950 the majority of staphylococcal infections in hospitals throughout the world were penicillin-resistant.

As discussed in Chapter 7, staphylococci have achieved this by certain of them having the ability to secrete an enzyme known as penicillinase which destroys penicillin. In 1940 the number of such strains was extremely few, but gradually over the years with the destruction of strains sensitive to penicillin they have become increasingly numerous. It is important to understand that this enzyme, chemically a beta-lactamase, is not some protective device recently invented by certain strains of staphylococci since coming under attack by penicillin, as there is good evidence that both these and other organisms have been producing this substance for a very long time. M. Segalove has reported that a strain of *Staphylococcus* capable of synthesizing this enzyme was isolated from a food poisoning outbreak in Omaha in 1932. And what is even more fascinating, P. H. A. Sneath of the National Institute of Medical Research in London, writing in *Nature* in 1962, describes how recent examination of soil samples taken from around plant specimens collected in the sixteenth century and stored in the British Museum has yielded strains of an organism known as *Bacillus licheniformis*, the spores of which contain large amounts of penicillinase.

The discovery that the genes for penicillinase production are not only replicated in every daughter cell but can be passed from one cell to another by viruses known as bacteriophages, was made by H. L. Ritz and J. M. Baldwin working at the Ohio State University in 1958, but it was not until 1963 that Richard Novick working at the

Rockefeller Institute in New York showed that these genes are not contained in the chromosomes but in separate DNA-containing structures known as plasmids.

During the early 1950's the fact that penicillin was no longer effective against staphylococci found in hospitals did not at first seem to be a matter for concern, as by that time several other suitable antibiotics had become available including streptomycin, chloramphenicol, the tetracyclines, erythromycin and novobiocin. However the fairly rapid emergence of strains of this organism resistant to all these antibiotics, with some carrying their resistance 'know-how' in chromosomes and others in plasmids, quickly cast a threatening shadow on the horizon. Fortunately by then bacteriologists had come to recognize that by withdrawing an antibiotic for a time the number of strains resistant to it would diminish sufficiently for it once again to become useful. One of the first to put this principle into practice was Mark Ridley, the microbiologist at St Thomas's Hospital, London, who, finding in 1958 that 18 per cent of staphylococci isolated from patients in that hospital had become resistant to all the available antibiotics, suggested to his clinical colleagues that all prescribing of erythromycin and novobiocin should be temporarily forbidden. Although this meant the suppression of individuals' clinical freedom, this policy was adopted with the result that in a matter of only a few months the number of strains resistant to these two antibiotics had fallen to such a low level as to make their use profitable once again. It was generally realized that such a manoeuvre could only be but a temporary expedient and that there was an urgent need for the pharmaceutical industry to discover some new drugs, and everyone concerned was therefore very relieved when Beecham Research Laboratories in 1960 announced the discovery of methicillin, the first semi-synthetic penicillinase-resistant penicillin.

The introduction of other powerful anti-staphylococcal agents, including fucidin in 1960, the replacement of methicillin by cloxacillin in 1961, the discovery of lincomycin in 1962, gentamicin in 1963, various cephalosporins from 1964 onwards and the replacement of lincomycin by clindamycin in 1967 and of cloxacillin by flucloxacillin in 1970, not unreasonably led to the hope that the *Staphylococcus* might before long be brought under permanent control, but once again the emergence of strains resistant first to one and then another of these agents has removed any prospect of this occurring within the foreseeable future.

It is therefore sad to relate that the excitement experienced in the early 1940's, when life-threatening staphylococcal infections were readily cured by penicillin, was soon to be replaced, once it was found that this organism was becoming increasingly penicillin-resistant, by a spirit of disillusionment which more than thirty years later and in spite of the discovery of a large number of other powerful anti-staphylococcal drugs has still to be dispelled.

The other group of bacteria which because of their special aptitude for developing resistance to anti-microbial agents are causing much trouble, are the Gram-negative bacilli known collectively as the Enterobacteriaceae (p. 37). These bacilli have learned how to pass on to each other various types of genetic information including the capacity for drug resistance, by pairs of cells undergoing conjugation. During this process male or donor cells attach themselves to female or recipient cells by means of hair-like appendages known as sex pili, and then transfer to the female cells DNA-containing transmissible plasmids. This type of activity has led some people to refer some-what imprecisely to the sex life of Gram-negative bacilli! But it should however be made clear that conjugation plays no part in the reproduction of these bacteria, unlike what happens in the more conventional sex act practised by higher forms of life. The mating that takes place between these bacteria, resulting in the transfer of DNA material from a male cell to a female one, immediately transforms the latter into a male! – enabling it to conjugate with other females. It is in this way that genetic information, including that relating to drug resistance, may rapidly spread through a population of enterobacteria.

It should be stressed that this method of exchanging genetic information takes place not only between bacteria of the same species but also between those of different species and, further, that resistance acquired in this manner is not usually just to one drug but rather to several at a time. This remarkable phenomenon, often referred to as 'infectious drug resistance', was first recognized

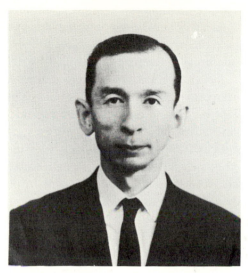

Fig. 61. Professor Tsutomu
Watanabe (1923–72).

during the later part of the 1950's in Japan and reported by Ochiai, Yamanaka, Kimura and Sawada in 1959 and by Akiba, Koyama, Ishiki, Kimura and Fukushima in 1960. It was in the same year that Mitsuhashi proposed that the transmissible agents responsible for this type of drug resistance should be known as resistance factors or 'R' factors, a term which has since been widely adopted.

All these various contributions to the subject appeared in Japanese journals and the Western world is indebted to Tsutomu Watanabe (1923–72) of the Keio University School of Medicine in Tokyo for bringing his compatriots' observations to the attention of English-speaking people by writing about this subject in the American *Bacteriological Reviews* in 1963. In his paper, entitled 'Infective Heredity of Multiple Drug Resistance in Bacteria', Watanabe also reports some of his own investigations carried out with financial assistance from the Ministry of Education of Japan and somewhat interestingly from the Waksman Foundation in that country.

It had been found from 1956 onwards in Japan that in outbreaks of bacillary dysentery whereas some strains of *Shigella* were sensitive to all the drugs currently in use, there was an increasing number of

other strains showing multiple resistance to the four drugs streptomycin, chloramphenicol, tetracycline and the sulphonamides; also,
that patients excreting drug-sensitive shigellae when treated with
only one of these drugs subsequently acquired organisms resistant
to all four of them. In 1959 Akiba ingeniously suggested that
Escherichia coli, an organism which is readily passed from one person
to another, might be playing an important part in spreading this
multiple drug resistance. Support for this idea was given by Ochiai
and his colleagues in 1959 and independently by Akiba and others
in 1960 when they were able to bring about transfer of resistance
from *Escherichia coli* strains to *Shigella* strains in the laboratory;
particularly when Mitsuhashi, Harada and Hashimoto in 1960
isolated strains of *Escherichia coli* with multiple resistance from
patients with bacillary dysentery. Since then it has been confirmed
by workers in all parts of the world that *Escherichia coli*, though
usually only a harmless commensal in the bowel, plays an important
part as an intermediary in the spreading of R factors to pathogenic
Escherichia and also to *Shigella*, *Salmonella*, *Klebsiella*, *Proteus* and
Pseudomonas organisms.

As the years have passed, R factors have appeared capable of
transmitting to these organisms resistance to most anti-microbial
drugs.

In 1963 R factors to kanamycin and neomycin were recognized by
G. Lebek amongst strains of *Salmonella typhimurium* responsible for
outbreaks of food poisoning in Germany. Since then they have been
reported from most parts of the world. Two years later in
Britain, E. S. Anderson and Naomi Datta identified R factors
capable of transmitting resistance to various penicillins, including
ampicillin and carbenicillin, and to the cephalosporins. During the
early 1970's R factors conferring on bacteria resistance to gentamicin
and trimethoprim have been discovered.

No R factor yet identified confers resistance to all these drugs
simultaneously; some only transmit resistance to one or two, but in
the majority it is to three, four, or even five drugs at a time and this
resistance is passed from one organism to another *en bloc*. As the
combination of drugs affected varies widely it is often possible to
recognize different R factors by the pattern of resistance they produce.

Some transmissible R factors arising in Gram-negative entero-bacteria exert their influence by altering the permeability of bacterial cell walls so as to impede the diffusion of antibiotics into bacteria. Others, by passing on certain genetic information, enable bacteria to produce enzymes capable of inactivating antibiotics. Included amongst these enzymes are various beta-lactamases capable of opening the lactam ring, an essential part of the structure both of the penicillins and the cephalosporins, with those acting against the penicillins often being referred to as penicillinases and those against the cephalosporins as cephalosporinases.

These enterobacterial penicillinases differ from staphylococcal penicillinase in so much that whereas the latter diffuses into the host's tissues destroying any penicillin or ampicillin in the neighbour-hood, those associated with Gram-negative organisms remain inside the bacteria destroying antibiotics as soon as they have penetrated their walls. Further, enterobacterial penicillinases are active not only against penicillin and ampicillin but also against the cephalosporins; this is in addition to the cephalosporinases present in certain enterobacteria which have a more specific destructive effect on cephalosporin antibiotics.

Finally there are other R factors which, by bringing about the release of enzymes such as phosphotransferase, adenylsynthetase and acetyltransferase, inactivate streptomycin and other related antibiotics by interfering with the biochemistry of these substances whilst leaving their structure intact.

The rapid increase in incidence of the spread of R factors since they were first identified in Japan in the 1950's has been alarming. In Japan during 1955 amongst *Shigella flexneri*, the main cause of bacillary dysentery in that country, only one strain was found to possess an R factor carrying resistance to streptomycin, tetracycline, chloramphenicol and the sulphonamides. By 1970, 70 per cent of strains possessed this factor. Dr Joan Davies and her colleagues who in London have studied the *Shigella sonnei*, the cause of the much milder form of bacillary dysentery seen in Britain, have observed much the same pattern of events. A few multiple resistant strains of this organism first appeared in the late 1950's, but by 1970 70 per cent of strains had become resistant to at least three drugs.

The incidence of R factors in *Salmonella* found in Great Britain has been studied by E. S. Anderson, and those in Holland by A. Manten and his colleagues. In both countries the incidence has rapidly increased from about 2 per cent at the beginning of the 1960's to about 60 per cent by the mid 1960's.

The fact that in this country most *Salmonella* food poisoning organisms and *Shigella sonnei* dysentery organisms are now resistant to treatment with antibiotics is not of particular importance in itself, as in both cases the infection is mild and there is no necessity for antibiotic treatment except in the occasional case when the infection spreads outside the bowel. However what is of great concern is that these resistant organisms are capable of transmitting multiple drug resistance to other bacteria in the bowel, such as *Escherichia coli*, which in turn may not only be the cause of drug-resistant disease themselves but may convey this drug resistance to other Gram-negative species.

Human infection with *Salmonella typhimurium* is usually the result of food poisoning and it would seem that the main reservoir of infection is farm animals including pigs, chickens and calves. E. S. Anderson and his colleagues working at the Enteric Reference Laboratory in London first drew attention to this when they studied outbreaks of *Salmonella typhimurium* enteritis amongst calves in Britain during 1963-6. They thought that the spread of infection was encouraged by the animals being taken from farms and herded together in large numbers in huge rearing centres which were both unhygienic and overcrowded. Large amounts of one or other antibiotic used in an attempt to control the outbreaks of diarrhoea in these animals only resulted in an increasing proportion of *Salmonella typhimurium* strains acquiring resistance to several antibiotics at a time, with the R factors responsible for this multiple resistance being found not only in the offending *Salmonella* organisms but also in the commensal *Escherichia coli* in these animals. These workers were then disturbed to find that such outbreaks were paralleled by a rise in incidence of human food poisoning due to the identical organism carrying the same R factors.

Prior to the introduction of antibiotics, bacterial infection was the cause of serious losses in livestock and there can be no argument that

farmers have derived much benefit from giving animals these substances. They have not always administered them wisely. For example,
sometimes when infection breaks out on a farm an antibiotic is given
in a blunderbuss manner to all the animals in the hope that it will
cure those that are ill and prevent the infection from spreading to
those that are fit. Even worse is when there is no infection on a farm
and yet healthy animals are given small amounts of an antibiotic
prophylactically on a long-term basis. Unfortunately such misuse of
antibiotics only encourages the formation of R factors, their spread
amongst Gram-negative organisms in these animals' intestines and
their eventual transfer from these animals to man. Similarly the
practice of giving small amounts of penicillin or tetracycline to young
animals in food supplements in order to stimulate their growth also
encourages the development of R factors capable of spreading
resistance to these antibiotics in the intestinal organisms in these
animals, and for these R factors in turn to be passed on to man.

Concern about these matters in Great Britain led to the setting up
of a Committee under Professor Swann which submitted its Report
to Parliament in 1969. In this Report the Committee recommend
that the use of penicillin and tetracycline for growth promotion
should cease and that they should be replaced for this purpose by
antibiotics which are not in use in the treatment of disease in cattle
or man. The replacements approved by the Committee include
bacitracin, virginiamycin and flavomycin. In addition they recommend that the full range of antibiotics used in man should be
available for treating disease in cattle but that they should only be
prescribed, and their administration supervised by members of the
veterinary profession.

A serious consequence of the spread of R factors resulting from
the indiscriminate use of antibiotics can be seen in various parts of
the world where in epidemics of typhoid fever the causative *Salmonella
typhi* organism has recently been found to be resistant to chloramphenicol. This is particularly tragic because since chloramphenicol was first discovered in the early 1950's it has remained the
antibiotic of choice for this particular disease and once its importance
in this respect had been recognized its use in the treatment of all
other more commonly occurring infections should have been dis-

continued, especially as by that time other suitable alternatives for treating these, including the tetracyclines, were available. Somewhat paradoxically it was fortunate that in many parts of the world its occasional but nevertheless serious effects on the bone marrow (p. 151) did eventually lead to its use in the treatment of routine infections being discontinued, as this has greatly reduced the chances of resistance to it spreading amongst bacteria, and allowed it to be kept in reserve for the treatment of typhoid fever, a disease whose dangers when untreated far outweigh any potential risk from the side effects of this antibiotic. In certain countries however doctors have continued to prescribe it for a variety of conditions and worse still the general public have been allowed to buy it over the counter without a prescription, with the result that it is often taken for inadequate reasons and in sup-optimal amounts. Such large-scale use and even abuse of this antibiotic has inevitably encouraged the spread of resistance to it in intestinal bacteria and in places where typhoid fever is endemic it was only a matter of time before R factors carrying resistance to this drug appeared in strains of *Salmonella typhi*. It was precisely for these reasons that in Mexico in 1972 a chloramphenicol-resistant strain of *Salmonella typhi* appeared, causing more than 10,000 cases of typhoid fever with a number of foreign visitors to that country being affected, including at least fifty-two Americans, two British, and one Swiss, all of whom were capable of spreading the disease on returning to their own country. Similar chloramphenicol-resistant epidemics have been reported in India, Vietnam and Thailand. As E. S. Anderson says in his paper 'The Problem and Implications of Chloramphenicol Resistance in the Typhoid Bacillus', published in the *Journal of Hygiene* in 1975, 'The time has clearly come when international cooperation at legislative and professional levels is needed to attempt to reverse the change in the ecology of the enterobacteria and other organisms that has resulted from the indiscriminate use of antibacterial drugs.'

Naomi Datta, who has done so much important work in unravelling the mysteries of transmissible antibiotic resistance in disease has also, with her colleagues at the Royal Postgraduate Medical School in London, studied the incidence of R factors in bacteria in the faeces of healthy people. They have found that about 50 per cent of adults in the general community harbour R factors in their intestinal bacteria and that in about 30 per cent these R factors are present in large numbers. Datta also has found that the drugs to which the normal bowel bacteria are most often resistant are streptomycin, tetracycline and the sulphonamides, and further that admission to hospital has only a slight effect in increasing the number of R-factor-carrying bacteria. Others have shown that R factors are carried even more frequently by normal babies and young children.

Datta's observations on the effects of oral administration of antibiotics are interesting. Somewhat surprisingly she found that oral administration of ampicillin or sulphonamides did not cause much rise in the incidence of R factors but that a course of tetracycline led to the excretion of *Escherichia coli* resistant not only to tetracycline but also to ampicillin, streptomycin, chloramphenicol and the sulphonamides. It is fortunate however that R factors disappear within weeks or months of an antibiotic being used, as otherwise resistance to all the commonly used antibiotics would by now have rendered them completely useless.

Urinary tract infections arising in people in the general community are in 80 per cent of the cases due to *Escherichia coli*, with the remainder being due to *Proteus mirabilis*. In infections acquired in hospital, in addition to these Gram-negative organisms other Gram-negative ones including species of *Proteus*, *Klebsiella*, and *Pseudomonas aeruginosa*, together with the Gram-positive *Streptococcus faecalis*, may be responsible. The spread of R factors throughout the whole range of these Gram-negative organisms means that antibiotic resistance in urinary tract infections, particularly those acquired in hospitals, is widespread and unpredictable. Fortunately the large number of antimicrobial agents now available for treating such infections, including the sulphonamides, ampicillin, amoxicillin, the cephalosporins, nalidixic acid, nitrofurantoin, co-trimoxazole, cycloserine, kanamycin, streptomycin, carbenicillin and gentamacin, mean that for infections in general practice there are usually several drugs from which to choose and in the treatment of the more intractable hospital-acquired infections there is fortunately usually still at least one antibiotic to which the organisms are sensitive.

As long ago as 1959, Maxwell Finland and his colleagues writing in the *Journal of the American Medical Association* drew attention to the fact that the introduction and widespread use of anti-microbial agents had been associated with a striking increase in the incidence of infections due to staphylococci and enterobacteria resistant to these drugs. This state of affairs has since been confirmed many times and is due to the abundant use of antibiotics in the enclosed environments of hospitals causing sensitive strains of organisms to be destroyed and for their place to be taken by a proliferation of resistant ones, some being sensitive strains which have become resistant whilst others have been resistant from the start.

The implication of this is that paradoxically the hospital environment which was always susceptible to the spread of serious infection before the advent of Listerean antisepsis has, since the introduction of modern antibiotics, once again become the breeding ground of virulent organisms. The enterobacteria concerned in the everyday spread of infection in hospitals include *Escherichia coli, Klebsiella,* and *Proteus,* all of which because of a steady increase in transmissible resistance have become difficult to combat, and in addition *Pseudomonas,* an organism which has always had a high degree of natural resistance.

These organisms are not only the cause of patients in hospital acquiring troublesome urinary tract infections but also are often the cause of sepsis in accidental wounds, surgical wounds and burns and at times of life-threatening pneumonia, meningitis and septicaemia.

The realization that certain patients in hospital whose resistance to infection is lowered as a result of serious disease may be attacked by such organisms, not unreasonably led to them being given antibiotics in an attempt to prevent this from happening. This prophylactic use of antibiotics only made the situation worse, for all it succeeded in doing was to kill off sensitive organisms in such people and for those to be replaced by resistant ones from the environment. This was well illustrated by the course of events in a neurosurgical unit in Britain where, because in 1966 there was an increasing incidence of post-operative wound sepsis due to infection with staphylococci and enterobacteria, a number of patients were given ampicillin and cloxacillin in an effort to avoid this complication. The result of this was that whilst bacteria sensitive to these antibiotics were eradicated, highly virulent *Klebsiella* took their place so that between October 1968 and May 1969 out of 228 patients admitted to the intensive care section of the unit this highly dangerous organism was the cause of pneumonia in approximately one out of every three patients, of urinary tract infection in one out of every five, and of meningitis in seven patients. An attempt between July and September 1969 to attack this organism aggressively with exceptionally large amounts of a suitable antibiotic benefited individual patients but made no difference to the number of organisms in the environment. Faced with the possible closure of the unit all concerned accepted the advice of the bacteriologist to stop using all antibiotics both prophylactically and therapeutically from October 1969 to January 1970. The result of this was that the dreaded *Klebsiella* rapidly disappeared and what perhaps is even more remarkable is that no patient appears to have come to harm through lack of treatment with an antibiotic! Since that time the use of antibiotics in the unit has been strictly reserved for the treatment of a limited number of life-threatening infections.

It is as a result of this and other similar experiences that the use of antibiotics to protect hospital patients from infection with the many bacteria which surround them in the environment has for the most part been discontinued. Instead, special importance is placed on preventing cross infection, by the staff strictly adhering to accepted rules of hygiene, by the isolation of highly infectious patients and probably most important of all by protecting vulnerable patients by placing them in preventive isolation.

Further, it cannot be overemphasized that both in hospitals and in the general community the incidence of drug resistance amongst bacteria is directly related to the degree to which antibiotics are used and for this reason it is now accepted that much constraint should be placed on their use. The general public should learn not to expect to be given antibiotics for every febrile illness unless there is good reason to believe that the illness is of bacterial origin and furthermore is of such severity that it cannot be overcome by the body's natural defences.

It therefore can be seen in our continuing battle against bacteria that whilst there has been remarkable progress in the discovery of powerful anti-microbial agents, the enemy has become increasingly skilful both in defending itself against their action and in actively attacking them. Whilst rightfully giving praise to all those who have been and continue to be engaged in the development of such substances, let us not forget the important contributions made by those in the field of public health whose various achievements, including the control of vector insects and the development of prophylactic vaccines, have also done so much to keep the battle running in our favour up to now.

This having been said there can be no doubt that the discovery of antibiotics has been, and continues to be, an enormous blessing to mankind. Many erstwhile disabling and at times lethal bacterial diseases may now be cured so that countless people can be relieved of much suffering and by defying death in the earlier periods of life are enabled to complete their natural span of years. In the affluent countries of the world this happy state of affairs has however contributed to the natural process of selection being upset and this in turn has in part been responsible for birth control becoming so essential. These various factors put together are resulting in an increasing proportion of elderly people being supported by a relatively decreasing number of those of working age. This situation, with its important economic and sociological implications will become even more accentuated when at some time in the future efficient cytotoxic drugs for combating cancer are discovered. Such considerations, far from being a cause for concern, should be a challenge to society to see that the benefits conferred on it by modern science are not replaced by the miseries associated with a mounting tide of loneliness in old age.

INDEX OF NAMES

SUBJECT INDEX

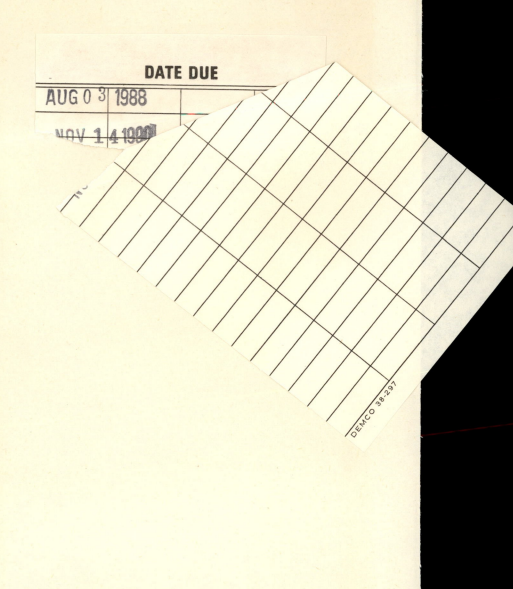